Sasang Constitutional Medicine and Clinical Application

Sasang Constitutional Medicine and Clinical Application

This Edition was published by Jipmoondang in 2019, Seoul, Korea.

Jipmoondang
5th Floor, 82 Donhwamun-ro, Jongno-gu, Seoul, 03134, Korea
Phone: +82-1811-7567
E-mail: sale@jipmoon.com
Homepage: www.jipmoon.com

The National Library of Korea Cataloging-in-Publication (CIP)
Sasang Constitutional Medicine and Clinical Application
Seoul, Korea: Jipmoondang, 2019
ISBN 978-89-303-1821-1 93510 519.74-KDC6 616.075-DDC23
CIP2019013066

Printed in Korea

Sasang Constitutional Medicine and Clinical Application

Koh Byung Hee

JIPMOONDANG

Congratulatory address

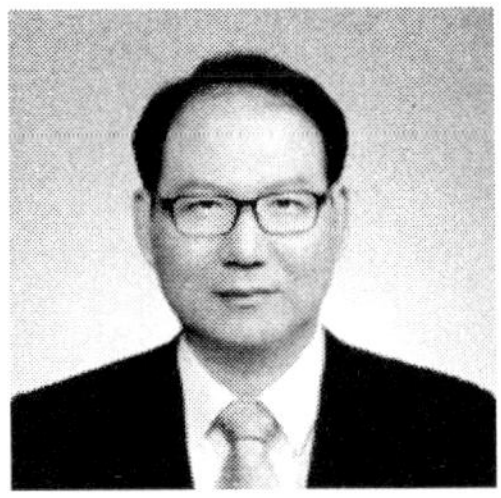

As an honorary president of the Society of Sasang Constitutional Medicine and a former head of KIOM(Korea Institute of Oriental Medicine), Prof. Koh, Byung Hee is a very important figure in the field of Korean medicine.

Prof. Koh has been making unceasing efforts to spread Korean medicine and Sasang constitutional medicine worldwide by participating in various international academic conferences and having chaired in an international conference for standardizing Korean medicine terminologies.

Endeavoring to well-promote Sasang constitutional medicine to foreigners, this book was published by gathering pieces of writings he wrote from the sense of necessity towards a book that can promote and educate Sasang constitutional medicine to foreigners.

In terms of organization, the contents are ordered in a way that can be easily understood by people learning Sasang constitutional medicine: the meaning of Sasang constitutional medicine, Dr. Lee Jema, Sasang constitution diagnosing methods, Sasang constitution acupuncture methods, application of Sasang constitutional medicine by disease types, and constitutional regimens by constitution types.

The contents of the book are also composed of sentences and terms that are understandable considering that its target readers are foreigners who are unfamiliar with Sasang constitutional medicine.

In 'Donguisusebowon', Dr. Lee, Jema states that all persons possess specialties of their own, such as good writing skills, fine archery or horse-riding skills, or skills for the game of go. As we all should develop our own specialties, Prof. Koh, Byung Hee seems to have a linguistic talent that supposedly indicate his specialty in introducing unfamiliar contents to foreigners.

I am very delighted that such a valuable book has been published amongst the reality where it is rare to find publications that introduce Sasang constitutional medicine in a foreign language. I hope that those who learn Sasang constitutional medicine will be able to grasp an understanding on Sasang constitutional medicine through this book, and use it as a tool to realize the excellency in Korean medicine. It will be proven that Prof. Koh's great efforts have not been in vain, once the Sasang constitutional medicine is no longer confined to Korea, but becomes a cosmopolitan Sasang constitutional medicine on a global level. Thank you.

T. S. Yu

President, Yu, Junsang
Society of Sasang Constitutional Medicine

Recommendation

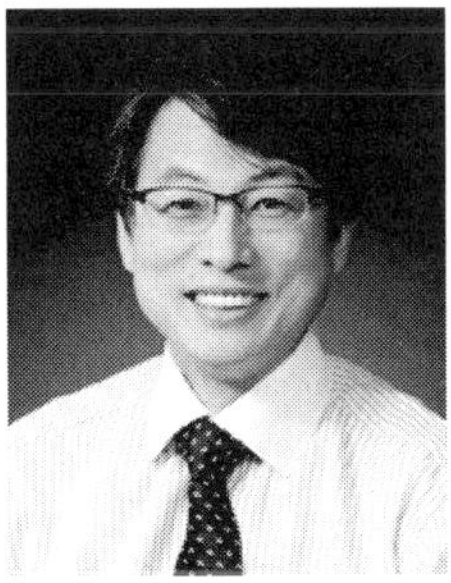

It gives me great pleasure to extend my congratulations on the publication of 《Sasang Constitutional Medicine and Clinical Application》, which will be a messenger promoting the excellence of the Sasang Constitutional Medicine (SCM) all over the world.

Traditional medicines of different countries have changed and developed in numerous varied ways sharing the rise and fall of relevant peoples. Some of the leading examples are traditional Korean medicine, traditional Chinese medicine and Ayurveda from India, but only a small number of them are still widely used clinically and studied systematically.

SCM, a theoretical system representing the originality of Korean medicine, is a unique traditional medical model that divides people's physical constitutions into four types and offers traditional medical treatment suitable for each constitutional type. Lee, Jema, a Confucian scholar and medical scientist in the Late Joseon Dynasty, first introduced SCM in his book 《Donguisusebowon》. According to him, people were divided into four constitutional types based on body shape, personalities, symptoms, etc., and different medications and remedies were needed to effectively treat people who belonged to different constitutional types even though they had the same symptoms. As such, Korean medicine borne out of our ancestors' wisdom, and in particular SCM, have practiced personalized medicine based on the constitutional types of individuals since the late 19th century.

It is also a field of medicine that perfectly matches the direction being sought by the future medicine. The appropriate combination between ICT exemplified by AI, big data, mobile communications, etc. and SCM developed through the wisdom of our ancestors will help expedite the realization of personalized medicine and preventive medicine for the future, which start with health management prior to the outbreak of diseases.

Although SCM is studied systematically and numerous research papers on the subject are being published in Korea, it is not widely known overseas. As a researcher of SCM, I have verified the possibility of applying it to people around the world other than Koreans through the collaborative efforts with professionals in such countries as China, Japan, and Vietnam.

I hope that the book will contribute to broadening the understanding and clinical application of Korea's SCM by scholars, clinicians, and researchers in traditional medicine as well as complementary and alternative medicine throughout the world, and anticipate that it will present a great opportunity to appreciate Lee, Jema's philosophy and experiences that he handed down to us more than 100 years ago.

Thank you.

김종열

May 2019

Kim, Jongyeol, KMD, Ph.d.

President

Korea Institute of Oriental Medicine

Forward

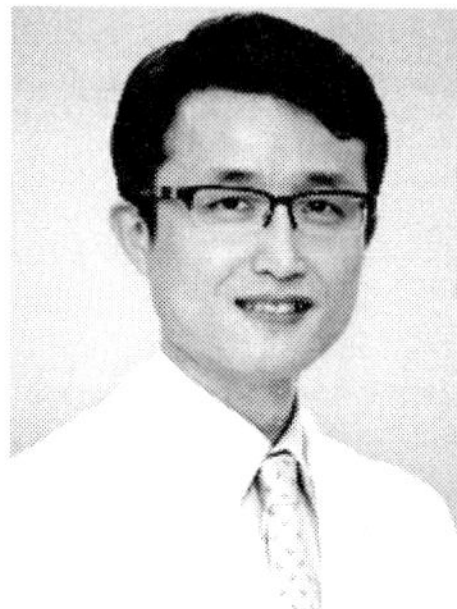

I extend my heartiest congratulations on Prof. Byunghee Koh's publication, "Sasang Constitutional Medicine and Clinical Application."

Prof. Koh is the leading expert on Sasang Constitutional Medicine (SCM) based on his vast research and publications utilizing SCM to treat patients with various diseases and disorders. He has brought tremendous international attention regarding the true medical benefits of SCM on a global scale.

Korea has established its own medical sciences and traditional medicine techniques and SCM is one form of practice of Korean medicine developed by Dr. Jema Lee about 120 years ago. Generally speaking, practitioners of SCM, such as Prof. Koh, believe that all individuals have their own bodily "constitution" and that a doctor should treat and write prescriptions according to such constitutions. Such a belief is a shift from standard traditional Asian medicine practices originating from China and SCM practitioners have documented vast clinical cases in which novel medicines based on this fundamental paradigm have been truly effective.

There is no question that the use and application of SCM, integrative medicine, and acupuncture are on the rise in all parts of the world, as more and more clinical studies and the exposure of these new alternative methods are becoming more commonplace.

Prof. Koh is the ultimate resource in the field and he has made it his mission to spread the value of SCM around the world. I believe that this excellent book will play a significant role in bridging the gap between the Western and Eastern treatment methods. It will act as a catalyst to generate more scholarly interactions and acknowledgements between the two schools of medicine.

Again, I strongly recommend this book to not only relevant professionals but also lay public who are interested in maintaining their health and longevity by applying the healing art of SCM.

Thank you.

Best regards,

Sanghoon Lee, MD(Korean Medicine), MPH, PhD, Dipl.OM, LAc
Director, International Educational Institute of Korean Medicine
Professor, Acupuncture & Moxibustion, College of Korean Medicine
Vice-Director, WHO Collaborating Centre for Traditional Medicine
Kyung Hee University, Seoul, Republic of Korea

Acknowledgements

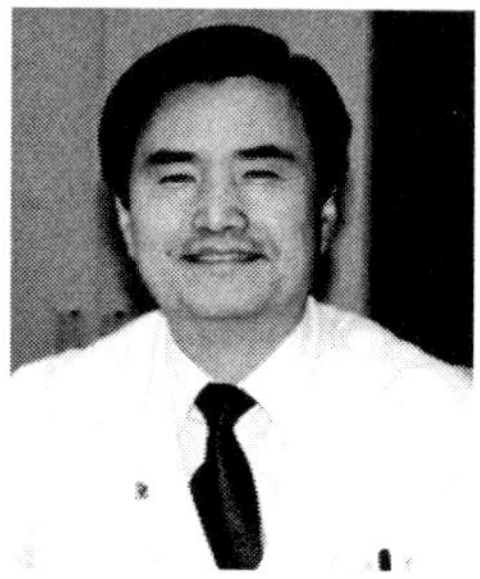

Sasang constitutional medicine is a representative theory of Korean medicine.

Founded by Dr. Lee, Jema, Sasang constitutional medicine has been handed down through exertions of many scholars including Prof. Hong, Soonyong, Prof. Roh, Jungwoo, Prof. Yom, Taehwan, Prof. Song, Ilbyung and many more. For more than 40 years since 1979, efforts have been made by the author for proper understanding and development of this field. In addition, dedication was made in the study through medical treatment with clinical application, research, and education.

As the society diversifies in terms of individual characteristics, differences of physical response to food and medicine, various mind control methods, and efficient harmonizing methods of social adaptation, Sasang constitutional medicine on therapeutic process and human relations will become even more influential. Considering that Dr. Lee, Jema informed us of such importance through Sasang constitutional medicine, this book can be of value to scholars and clinicians specializing this area.

Moreover, the IEIKM(International Education Institute of Korean Medicine in Kyunghee University) and the KIOM(Korea Institute of Oriental Medicine) have exerted every effort for the internationalization of Korean medicine. Developing textbooks that foreigners could easily access was what needed most improvement in the curriculum for foreigners. This book puts its basis on 'Sasang Constitutional Medicine' and 'New Compilation of Four Constitutional Medicine' that were published in cooperation with KIOM(Korea Institute of Oriental Medicine), and is supplemented with Acupuncture Treatment and Constitutional Regimens for clinical application from my article 'Clinical Application of Sasang Constitutional Medicine' in the book named 'Current practice of Korean Medicine', which was published in Pusan National University. I wish to express my sincere gratitude and appreciation to those who have contributed to the translation and publication of this book, including Prof. Song, Ilbyung, Prof. Lee, Euijoo, Prof. Lee, Sookyung, Prof. Lee, Junhee, Prof. Hwang, Minwoo and all hospital staff including Dr. Kang, Minsoo, Dr. Oh, Jiwon and Dr Lee, Hyeri, Dr. Lee, Jiwon and Dr. Kim, Hyunkoo who participated in translating, and Dr. Ahn, Sangwoo from the Institute, Prof. Lim, Byung mook, Ms. Jung, Hyunmi at Pusan National University. I also thank Mr. Lim, Donggyu for supporting the publication process of this book, as well as Ms. Jeon, Jeongah and Jang, Yiji for typesetting and proofreading the book from beginning to end.

Hopes are that clinicians as well as domestic and international scholars may gain more interest toward Sasang constitutional medicine from diverse areas through clinical application and research by using this book. In addition, I look forward to Sasang constitutional medicine, the tradition of Korean people, to develop into universal medicine that live through our lives.

Jungam(靜菴) Koh, Byung Hee
Department of Sasang Constitutional Medicine,
Kyunghee University Medical Center

Contents

- Congratulatory address / v
- Recommendation / vii
- Forward / ix
- Acknowledgements / xii

Understanding the Sasang Constitutional Medicine · 1

1. Sasang Constitutional Medicine 3
2. The influence of『Donguibogam』 6
3. Lee, Jema 8
4. The special qualities of Sasang Constitutional Medicine 13
5. Medicine that heals the mind 15
6. Constitutional Medicine of the past and present 17

Methods of differentiating Sasang Constitutions · 19

1. Constitutional typing based on physical appearances 23
   ① The Taeyang (TY) type 23
   ② The Soyang (SY) type 24
   ③ The Taeeum (TE) type 25
   ④ The Soeum (SE) type 26

2. Constitutional typing based on mental characteristics ········· 27
① The Taeyang (TY) constitutional type ········· 27
② The Soyang (SY) constitutional type ········· 29
③ The Taeeum (TE) constitutional type ········· 31
④ The Soeum (SE) constitutional type ········· 33
3. Constitutional typing based on pathological patterns ········· 35
① The Taeyang (TY) type ········· 36
② The Soyang (SY) type ········· 37
③ The Taeeum (TE) type ········· 38
④ The Soeum (SE) type ········· 39

Clinical Applications of Sasang Constitutional Medicine · 41

1. Constitution differentiation ········· 43
1) Sasang type differentiations based on appearance ········· 44
① Taeyangin ········· 44
② Soyangin ········· 44
③ Taeeumin ········· 44
④ Soeumin ········· 45
2) Constitution determinations based on mind and nature ········· 45
① Taeyangin ········· 45
② Soyangin ········· 46
③ Taeeumin ········· 46
④ Soeumin ········· 46
3) Constitution differentiations that are based on illness (病證) ·· 47
① Taeyangin ········· 47
② Soyangin ········· 48
③ Taeeumin ········· 48

④ Soeumin 48
2. Constitutional Illnesses 49
1) Illnesses that are prevalent in Taeyangin 49
2) Illnesses that are prevalent in Soyangin 50
3) Illnesses that are prevalent in Taeeumin 51
4) Illnesses that are prevalent in Soeumin 52
3. Acupuncture based on Sasang constitutions 54
1) Taekuk acupuncture method (太極鍼法) 54
2) Acupuncture based on constitution (體質針法) 54
4. Managing each Sasang type 55
1) Mind and body (心身) management 56
① Taeyangin 56
② Taeeumin 56
③ Soyangin 57
④ Soeumin 57
2) Nutrition for each Sasang type 57
① Taeyangin 58
② Taeeumin 58
③ Soyangin 59
④ Soeumin 59
3) Social life management for each Sasang type 60
① Taeyangin 60
② Soyangin 60
③Taeeumin 61
④ Soeumin 61
Appendix: Sasang Constitution Questionnaire 64
How to evaluate the results 71

Symptomatological Collection of Prescriptions in Korea's Sasang Medicine · 73

1. Symptomatological Collection of Prescriptions in Korea's Sasang Medicine 東醫四象用藥彙分 75
1) Wind 75
2) Cold 78
3) Summerheat 82
4) Dampness 83
5) Dryness 83
6) Fire 84
7) Internal damage 84
8) Consumptive Disease 86
9) Cholera and Gastroenteritis 86
10) Cough 87
11) Aggregation-Accumulation 88
12) Puffy Swelling 91
13) Distention and Fullness 91
14) Wasting-Thirst 92
15) Jaundice 93
16) Malaria 93
17) Mental Derangement 94
18) Essense 94
19) Qi 95
20) Spirit 97
21) Blood 98
22) Voice 100
23) Fluid and humor 101
24) Phlegm-Retained Fluid 101

25) Worm 103
26) Urine 104
27) Stool 105
28) Head 107
29) Face 108
30) Eyes 108
31) Ear 109
32) Nose 110
33) Mouth and Tongue 111
34) Teeth 111
35) Throat 112
36) Chest 113
37) Breast 113
38) Abdomen 114
39) Waist 115
40) Hypochondrium 115
41) Skin 115
42) Upper Limbs 115
43) Lower Limbs 116
44) Anterior Yin 116
45) Posterior Yin 117
46) Abscess and Carbuncle 117
47) Various Abscess 118
48) Gynecology and Obstetrics 118
49) Pediatrics 121
Sasang Formulas and Prescriptions 東醫四象新編劑方 125

Daily Health Maintenance using Sasang Constitutional Theory · 205

1. Beneficial and Harmful Foods 208
① The Taeyang (TY) type 211
② The Soyang (SY) type 212
③ The Taeeum (TE) type 212
④ The Soeum (SE) type 213
2. Preserving health by exercising adequate mental control .. 213
3. Appropriate Exercises 219

Curriculum Vitae 221
bibliography 223
Index 255

Understanding the Sasang Constitutional Medicine

1. Sasang Constitutional Medicine

Sasang Constitutional Medicine is a medical tradition that studies the physiological and pathological traits of the four constitutional types, namely the Taeyang (TY) type, Soyang (SY) type, Taeeum (TE) type, and Soeum (SE) type. The concept that constitution can be "typed" is the most basic underlying paradigm evident in the 『Donguisusebowon』.

Lee, Jema's medical system is termed 'Constitutional Medicine' because it is rooted in the concept of constitutional typology, a unique methodology of typing people according to their constitutional makeup. His ideas were shaped in the 19th century, a time of much sociopolitical unrest. Perhaps influenced by the great social demand for change, the underlying philosophy observed in Constitutional Medicine is also unconventional with regards to the traditional confucianist beliefs.

『Donguisusebowon』 was written after the completion of 『Gyeokchigo』. In the book, he continues to expand on his ground- breaking ideas. Constitutional Medicine does not revolve around the Yin Yang theory or the Meridian System theory as did the conventional medicine, but rather concentrates on the type of constitution, explaining the physiology, pathology, and treatment and prevention of disease particular to each constitutional type.

Lee, Jema's works reveal the new medical paradigms he discovered while studying conventional medicine. They also mention the medical figures and written works that had influenced him the most.

Knowledge of the people and works that contributed to the shaping of his theories can help us understand Constitutional Medicine better, and one of the people he had held in high esteem was Zhang Zhongjing.

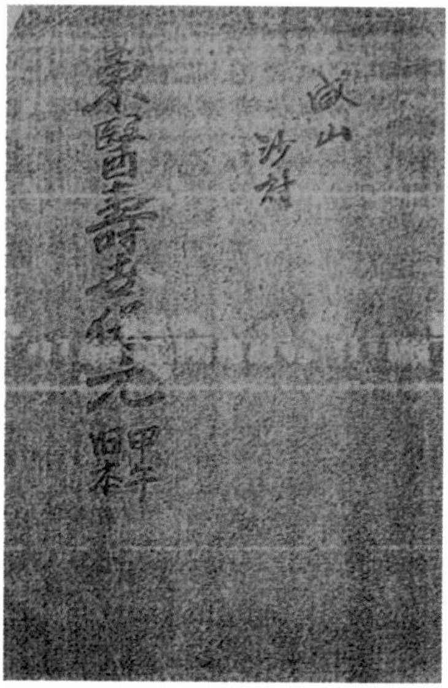

Donguisusebowon Gabo edition

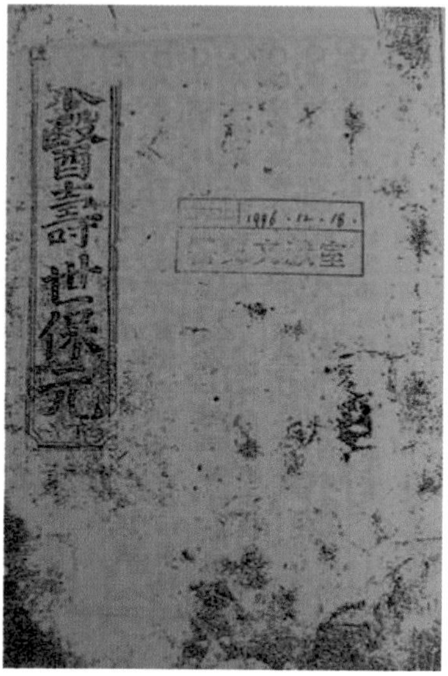

Donguisusebowon Sinchuk edition

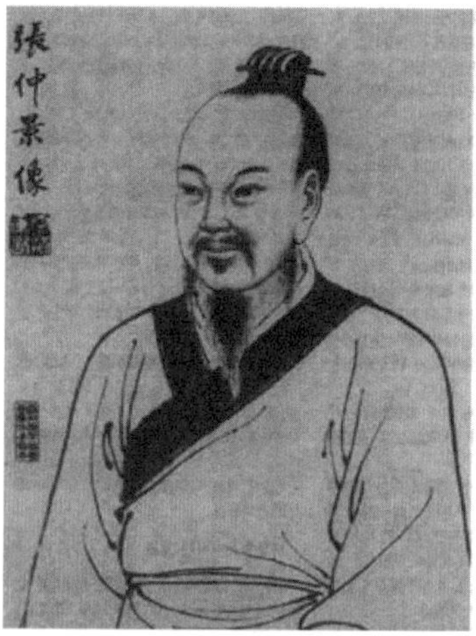

Zhang Zhongjing

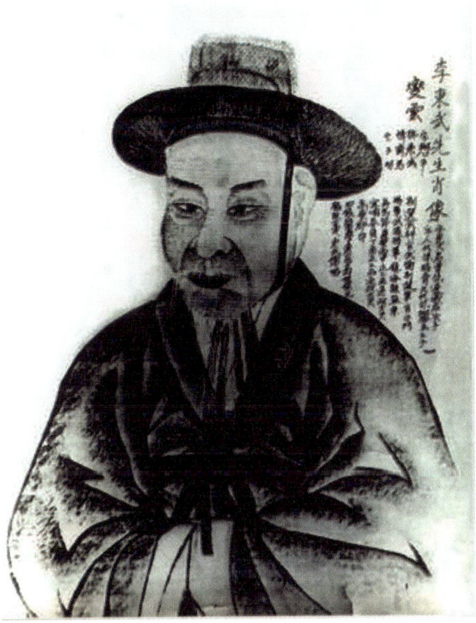

Dongmu Lee, Jema

For background information, He was the author of the classic script 『Shanghanlun』. 『Huangdi Neijing』,[1] the archetypical book from which all of traditional medicine had stemmed, proposes imbalance within the body and disharmony with nature as the most im-

1) **『Huangdi Neijing』**
Also called Neijing. It is narrated in a dialogue between Huangdi (a mythical ruler of China), the purported author, and Gi-baek (a retainer at the royal court), but historians agree that the real author had burrowed these historical figures for namesake only. The work consists of 18 books, divided into two volumes nine books each which are each titled "Suwen" and "Lingshu". Suwen explains the natural laws in traditional medicine, such as the Law of Harmony Between Man and Nature and the Law of Yin and Yang, but does not contain the actual clinical procedures. Lingshu contains material on acupuncture and moxibustion, but gives little explanation on herbal medicament. The surviving edition of Huangdi Neijing, annotated by Wang-bing in the Dang era, consists of twenty four books. There was also a thirty-book edition, edited by Yang-sang-seon in the Su era, that is no longer existent.

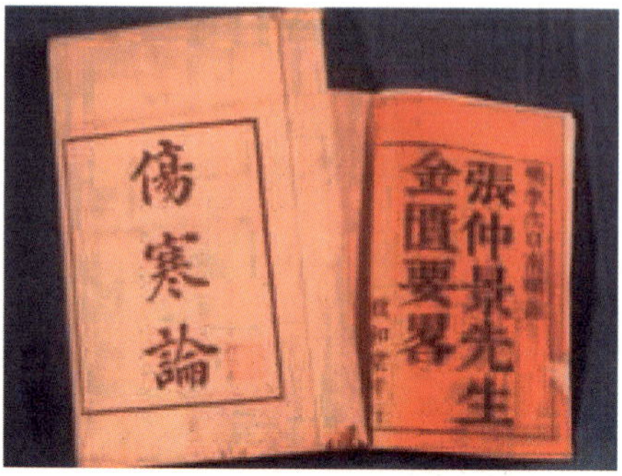

『Shanghanlun』

portant pathogenic factor; the book provided the most fundamental philosophical background for theories on the treatment and prevention of illnesses. On the other hand, 『Shanghanlun』 deals with the symptoms of and treatment for specific disorders; this book instructs more practical and detailed ways of treating patients.

Lee, Jema's medicine is more closely related to the 『Shanghanlun』 theories than those of 『Huangdi Neijing』, which suggests that he was more interested in the practical application of medicine. Most students of Constitutional Medicine follow this propensity and tend to focus more on the practical clinical application than on theoretical studies.

The important personage and books in the history of clinical medicine are quoted in various parts of 『Donguisusebowon』. Also mentioned are some of the writers whose works are often referred to by Lee, Jema. There is also a section introducing the respected physician Heo Jun and his ground breaking book, 『Donguibogam』.

2. The influence of 『Donguibogam』

Lee, Jema believed that the completion of 『Donguibogam』 marked

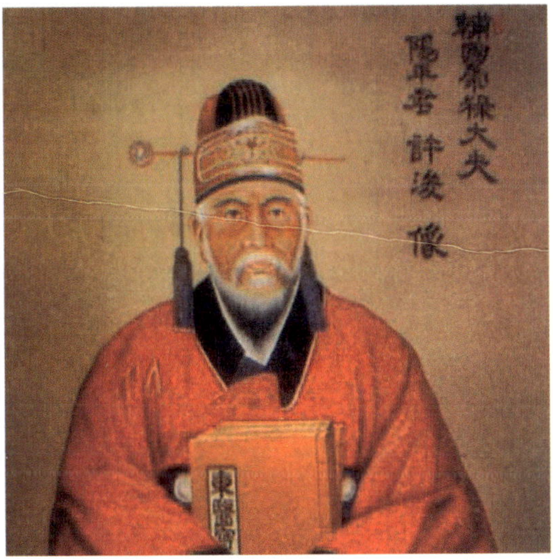

Heo Jun

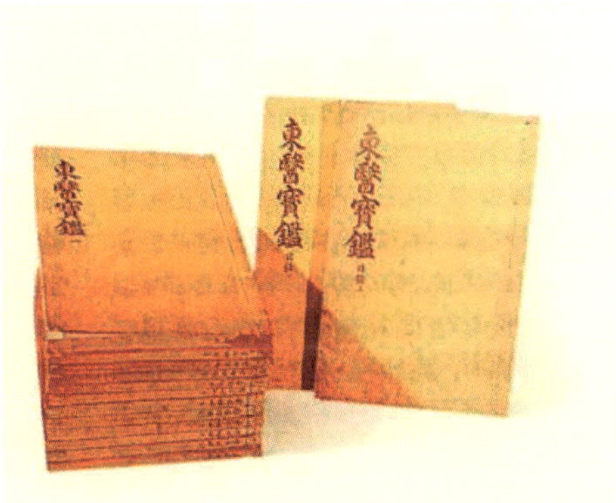

『Donguibogam』

the height of renaissance in Traditional Korean Medicine, and he paid the same respect to Heo Jun, the author, as he did to Zhang Zhongjing.

Lee, Jema refers to『Donguibogam』frequently in his writings, and the book clearly helped forge many of his theories.

He quotes passages from 『Donguibogam』 in his descriptions of pathological conditions, criticizing the conventional medical views and proposing new perspectives.

In his comments on preventive health care in 『Donguisusebowon』, he again burrows ideas from 『Donguibogam』, emphasizing Taoism and the importance role of moral integrity in leding a healthy life.

3. Lee, Jema

Lee, Jema (1837-1900) lived in the late Joseon dynasty. He was born in late 19th century and died at the break of 20th century. He lived through the "Period of the Riots" of the late 19th century and was one of the people who had experienced the upheavals of the society.

His given name was Dong-mu, and his appellation was Seop-wun or Seop-jin. His grandfather, Chung-won, and his father, Ban-oh, were descendents of the royal family, and Lee, Jema himself was the 19th descendent of Ahn-won Dae-gun, son of King Mok-jo. Lee, Jema was born on March 19, 1837 (on Korean lunar day), an illegitimate child of Ban-oh and his mistress.

There is an amusing anecdote about his birth. One day, Ban-oh visited a tavern and became heavily drunk. The owner of this tavern had a plain looking daughter of such difficult temperament that her parents could not find anyone to woo and marry her. When Ban-oh stayed for the night, the owner of the tavern furtively sent in his daughter to his room. Ten months later, Ban-oh's father dreamt of receiving one swift stallion from Jeju, an island famous for its highly reputed breed of horses. Days later, a woman came into his house with a baby in her arms, and the baby was thereafter named Je-ma (meaning 'horse of the Jeju Island').

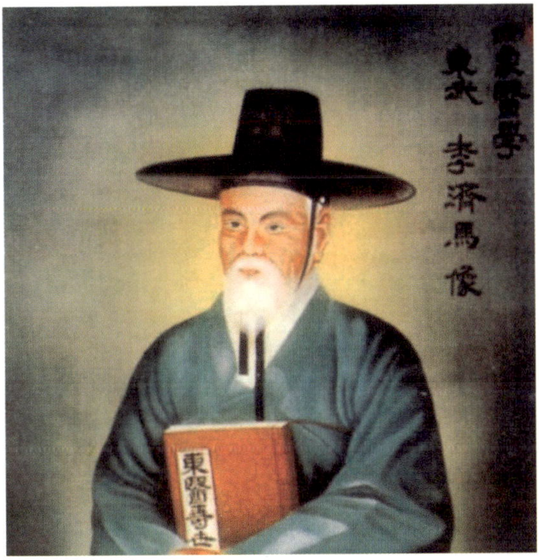

Lee, Jema

Although he was an illegitimate child, he was treated no differently from his siblings. He received excellent education and left influential works in philosophy and medicine. Above all, he discovered the Sasang Constitutional Medicine.

-. Governmental Post

Lee, Jema initially began his career in the military. He first became an official in 1875, at 39, and was promoted several times to different positions in the next eleven years.

In 1896, large scale riots led by Choe Mun-hwan stirred up nationwide disorder. Governmental intervention was on demand, and Lee, Jema was appointed head of the government force. He was again promoted in the following year, but retired in 1898.

In his prime, he mostly stayed near Hannamsan (or Hanbuksan), Gyeonggido. His mother became ill in 1895, precipitating his return to his birthplace. He opened a private clinic in his later years in Mansegyo, Hamheung.

-. Scholarly works

There are descriptions of Lee, Jema as strong-willed and decisive in temperament, and he won great love from his grandfather. A clever young man, he was educated by Jik-Jang, his uncle. He discovered his calling for martial arts and decided to pursue a military career. Not surprisingly, his given name "Dongmu" means "Warrior of the East."

He left home at the age of thirteen, travelling to faraway places to expand his experiences. In his youth, he travelled to Manchuria and the Soviet Union. He came across certain rare books in possession of a wealthy man named Hong, and it was there that he came in contact with the Western culture. Records tell us that, around 30, he chanced upon 『Myeongseonrok』, a book written by Han Seok-ji (1709-1803), which impacted him deeply.

Lee, Jema's philosophical viewpoints are revealed in a book of his, 『Gyeokchigo』.[2] The book contains of three chapters: 「Yuryak」, 「Banseong jam」, and 「Dokhaengpyeon」. 「Yuryak」, written between 1880 and 1889, attempts to reinterpret the classical confucianism within the frames of Sasang Constitutional Typology. 「Dokhaeng-pyeon」, written in 1882, proposes deeper knowledge and understanding of humanity as a solution for discord in relationships. 「Banseongjam」, written in 1893, expands on the same subject.

Lee, Jema's philosophical ideas essentially boil down to "understanding the human being and rectifying the self." This forms the groundwork for his proposition that the mind needs to be healed

2) 『Gyeokchigo』
This book best illustrates his philosophical groundwork in Sasang Constitutional Medicine. Here, he applied the Sasang philosophy, which pertains to the four phasic elements of natural phenomena, to explain both the cosmic mechanism and the human society. 『Donguisusebowon』 are together considered Lee, Jema's most representative works.

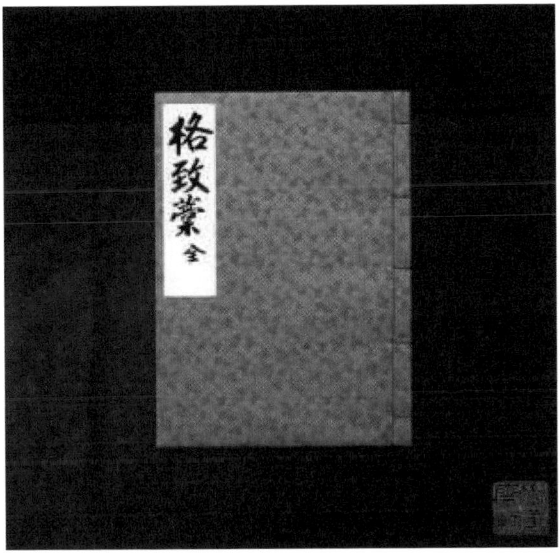

『Gyeokchigo』

in order to heal the body, expressed succinctly in the phrase "heal the mind to heal the body."

「Guangjeseol」 and 「Jejungsinpyeon」, writings on the preservation of health, and 『Dongmuyugo』, a recently rediscovered book, are all monumental works worthy of further study.

-. Medical studies

Lee, Jema himself had suffered from severe illnesses diagnosed as "Yeolgyeok (a set of symptoms characterized by emesis)" and "Haeyeok (a set of symptoms characterized by weakness of lower limbs)". This is probably one of the reasons he initially took interest in medicine. Otherwise there seems to have been no other means of educating himself on medicine.

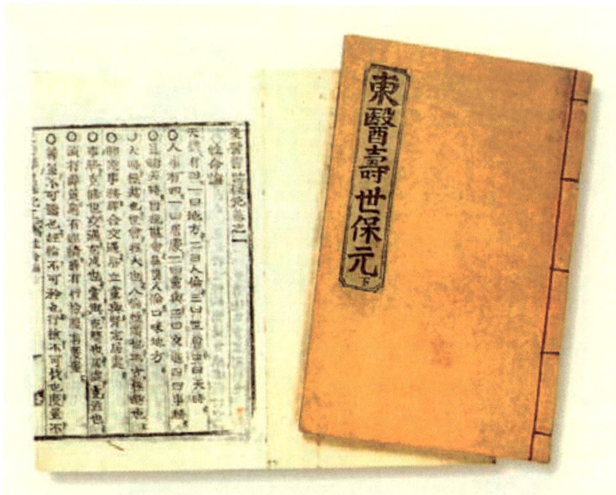

『Donguisusebowon』

There are passages in 『Donguisusebowon』[3)] that recount a successful treatment of the SY-type person using Yukmi-tang and Baekho-tang. Though he had not accumulated much experience at that time, the backbones of his theories were apparently under construction

---

3) **『Donguisusebowon』**

Pertains to the printed script containing 4 books in 2 volumes. Initially, only a part of the whole work was printed in 1894, and extended editions were printed afterwards. When Lee, Jema died in 1901, two of his students, Kim Yeong-gwan and Han Mok-yun, gathered the remaining material and published the final version.

This book contains the complete ideas on Sasang Constitution. It consists of seven chapters: 「Seongmyeong」, 「Sadan」, 「Hwakchung」, 「Jangbu」, 「Uiwon」, 「Gwangje」, and 「Sasangin byeongjeung」. Each chapter expounds on the clinical approach and the medicational system found in Sasang Constitutional Medicine. The book introduces a system of constitutional typology which categorizes people into four types of constitution (Taeyang type, Soyang type, Taeeum type, Soeum type). This medical system focuses on the constitutional type rather than on the manifest symptoms.

In contrast to the classical Traditional Korean Medicine, which has its roots in the Yin Yang and Five Elements theorem, Sasang Constitutional Medicine emphasizes the importance of the constitutional type. Medical historians view this shift of paradigm as a milestone in the history of medicine.

already.

He had started writing 『Donguisusebowon』 at the age of 57 in 1893 and completed it a year later, at the age of 58. He worked on a revised edition in 1899~1900, adding his by then extensive knowledge and experience. This book is considered the archetypical work in Sasang Constitutional Medicine because it lays the foundations of all the core concepts of the lore, explaining the physiology, pathology, pathophysiology, and treatment and prevention of disease for each constitutional type.

Recent excavation and rediscovery have come to show that Lee, Jema had written yet another book, 『Donguisusebowon』-Sasang chobongwon,[4] and scholars are investing great efforts in studying this work.

4. The special qualities of Sasang Constitutional Medicine[5]

The differences between conventional Traditional Korean Medicine

4) 『Donguisusebowon-Sasang chobongwon』
The author of this book remains yet to be determind, but specialists who have examined the text and the written style believe this script to be one of Lee, Jema's earlier works, written before 『Donguisusebowon』. It contains writings on his theoretical groundwork, preventive medicine, and the earlier Sasang Constitutional medicines.

5) The law of Yin and Yang states that the universe, both the microcosm and the macrocosm, is always composed of two contrasting sides, the Yin (Eum) and Yang—the dark and light, the cold and hot, the heavy and light. When this binary aspect is once again bifurcated, it results in the Sasang (四象), or the Four Reflections—the four aspects of a single phenomenon. The Yang (陽) bifurcates into Taeyang (太陽) and Soyang (少陽), and the Yin (陰), or Eum, into Taeeum (太陰) and Soeum (少陰). Lee, Jema's constitutional medicine is termed "Sasang Constitutional Medicine" because it is a system of constitutional typology that divides people into four types according to the constitutional makeup, namely Taeyang type (太陽人), Soyang type (少陽人), Taeeum type (太陰人), and Soeum type (少陰人).

and the Sasang Constitutional Medicine are as follows:

First, Sasang Constitutional Medicine sees each person as an individual with different constitutional traits.

Up till then, traditional medicine assumed that the physical body operates with the same mechanism for everyone. But in Constitutional Medicine, the four constitutional types respond differently to different situations, both physically and mentally. This gives rise to four distinct patterns of pathology and matching medications that are specific for each constitutional type. In the same contexts, medicational response is also different for each constitutional type. In other words, Sasang constitutional Medicine emphasizes the specific and unique pathological patterns found in each type of constitution.

Second, Sasang Constitutional Medicine is an idiosyncratic medicine.

Constitutional Medicine draws attention to the patient's idiosyncratic reaction to medication. Usually, patients do not respond uniformly to the same treatment. For one thing, eash person requires different amount of time for adequate treatment among people. The Yang types (Taeyang and Soyang types) respond quickly to medication, whereas the Eum types (Taeeum and Soeum types) require a longer period of time. Also, some constitutional types have greater propensity toward certain patterns of pathological progression. The Yangin tend to show a rapid disease progression, while the Eumin display a slower one. Therefore, it is necessary to take these factors into account and observe the idiosyncratic patterns.

Western therapy is generally centered around the "pathogen" part of illnesses. For example, when a patient is diagnosed pneumonia, he is treated with antibiotics that can exterminate the pathogenic agent. On the other hand, Eastern therapy focuses on the "host" part of illnesses. The causative agent is not directly dealt with, but rather the host is encouraged to recover and overcome the pathogenic factor on his own albeit with the help of therapeutic means. In other words, the pathogenic agent is indirectly incapacitated during treatment of the present symptoms. Furthermore, Sasang Constitutional Medicine provides specialized therapy for each constitutional type, which is why it can be called an "idiosyncratic" medicine.

Third, Constitutional Medicine asserts that the body is healed through healing of the mind.

According to constitutional traditional medicine, most illnesses fall into one of the two categories: disorders from external causes (eg. contagion, inclement weather, physical trauma) and disorders from internal causes (eg. unbalanced diet, unhealthy sex life). Sometimes, disorders from another pathogenic source (of much less significance is included): intemperate emotions and unfulfilled desires. In contrast, Lee, Jema perceived and emphasized the innate differences between the constitutional types that are rooted in the organ structural schemes of the body, or the structure of organ systems specific for each constitutional type. Even after birth, a person's physical conditions are constantly affected and forged by the mind. Therefore, controlling the mind is important for the prevention and treatment of disease. Each constitutional type has different desires and tendencies, which is why the mind is to be cultivated differently for different constitutional types.

5. Medicine that heals the mind

The Western medicine has advanced to the point where theoretically a person's life can be predicted and analyzed through genetic analysis. Moreover, Western medicine displays certain advantages over Eastern medicine; for example, Western medicine had discovered cure for cholera and smallpox, diseases which had killed so many in Korea in the Joseon dynasty.

Western medicine parted from natural philosophy in the late 18th century, and the breach of bondage perpetuates to this day. This was probably an inevitable event in the course of history, for the cultural current that had sprouted from mysticism and holism was how speeding toward scientism and rationalism.

But also, because the human being is composed of the mind as well as the body, medicine needs to embrace the psyche of the man. This demands a different perception that views the mind and body as two intricately interrelated elements of a homogeneous entity, a concept wholly different from the mind-body dualism paradigm prevalent in modern day Western medicine.

Morals and ethical standards are constructed as a culture is developed. Once the cultural worse is set, the members of the society adhere to the cultural standards without question, which is how the cultural code can: impact the society as a whole.

In case of Western medicine, the culture in which it is rooted lacks the close bondage between the sciences and philosophy that is required in order to understand the human psyche in a medical context. By contrast, the Eastern medicine, especially the Sasang Constitutional Medicine, had always retained close connections with the human psyche.

The virtues of this quality is not fully realized in today's society, possibly due to a lack of understanding of Eastern medicine and its consequent alienation from the predominant (Western) medicine. As proof, the Korean people mostly associate Korean Medicine with mystical herblore and natural remedies, at best visualizing it as a were form of preventive medicine. And so, further studies and efforts are required in order to promote Constitutional Medicine and to provide the public with a more comprehensive medical care.

6. Constitutional Medicine of the past and present

In the 19th century, Lee, Jema, a philosopher and a physician, proposed the Sasang Constitutional Typology and the relevant theories. The concepts he presented were based on the mainstream Confucianist doctrine in Joseon, and he also strived, as a medical practitioner, to provide the benefits of medicine as many people to as possible.

The foremost objective in his philosophy and medicine was to promote public well-being, of both mind and body, and to protect the general public from deadly epidemics. In 1894, his efforts culminated in the book Donguisusebowon, which underwent several revisions as more experience accumulated, until his death in 1900.

After his demise, his followers published a revised edition of the Donguisusebowon, which incorporated the first version (written in 1894) and the most recent one (completed in 1900). Han Dujeong, one of his students, printed the 7th edition in 1941, adding more herbal medications and presenting the material in a text simple enough for a layman to understand. In 1945, Choi Seung-dal and Lee Hyeon-jae established the Institute for Promotion of Sasang Constitutional Medicine. Hong Soon-yong and his followers launched the Society of Sasang Constitutional Medicine in 1970, setting off a full-scale research on Constitutional Medicine. Later in 1973, this organization officially became a subdivision of the Korean Oriental Medical Society. Regular meetings and conventions were held from 1979 onward. In 1989, the first issue of Journal of Constitutional Medicine was published, a journal that publishes basic theories, acupuncture, medication, preventive care, and scientific experiments relevant to Sasang Constitutional Medicine, now printing four issues each year. The Society of Sasang Constitutional Medicine has become the center for research on Sasang Constitutional Medicine for students, researchers, and practitioners alike.

Methods of differentiating Sasang Constitutions

The Three Criteria for Distinguishing Constitutions

In SCM(Sasang Constitutional Medicine) the three most important factors in differentiating constitutions are external appearance, mental characteristics and disease symptoms. External appearance is viewed in terms of the shape of the body and its countenance. Since each constitution has its own particular body shape, in many cases a constitution can be determined simply by looking at the shape of the body. The body will change over the course of a lifetime due to factors that influence physical growth such as nutrition and disease. In addition, exercise and physical habits can also influence the shape of the body. Nevertheless, the basic body shape remains unchanged. The ideas of body shape discussed in this chapter will give generalities about each constitutional type. However, because there are exceptions, it is not enough to only look at the shape of the body when identifying constitutions. One must also examine a person's mental characteristics.

Identifying constitutions by examining mental characteristics includes observing a person's temperament, talents, constant mental state (an innate state of mind maintained by a person of a given constitution throughout his or her lifetime – see the next section), personality, mental desire, etc. Each constitution has its own particular characteristics; therefore observing mental characteristics plays a great role in constitutional differentiation. It is, however, difficult to be objective when trying to identify one's own constitution. Although one might subjectively consider oneself to be an introvert, in reality it can be very difficult to objectively measure that characteristic. Also, there are some people who do not express their mental characteristics outwardly. In such cases, placing them in an unfamiliar situation and observing their reactions can be a means of determining their true mental nature.

Just as normal, healthy physiological conditions vary across each constitution, so do disease signs and symptoms. These disease manifestations can therefore be used to identify a particular constitution. The disease symptoms are first divided into mild and severe, but this division is not sufficient. Each constitution has a typical disease syndrome, but some constitutions show symptoms only when a disease is severe.

As we have seen, individual constitutions cannot be accurately identified using only a single criterion. Physical appearance, mental characteristics and disease symptoms must all be analyzed. While all three factors are important, if, after initial analysis, a person's constitution is not easily identifiable, his or her mental characteristics take precedence as the supreme determinant of constitution.

For reference, there was a recent attempt to relate Sasang constitutions to the four blood types (A, B, O and AB). It was hypothesized that there is a relationship between the four constitutions and the four blood types because they are both unchanging constitutional principles and because there are some differences in personality according to blood type. The theory posited that the TY type relates to AB blood type, TE-type to O, SE type to A, and SY type to B. Subsequent research showed no correlation between blood types and Sasang constitutions. Even though TY type is a rare constitutional type, there are many people who have AB blood. This alone indicates that the theory is flawed. There is also speculation that the Lewis blood group system has a considerable relationship with the Sasang constitutions although there has been no follow-up research.

Since interest in SCM is steadily increasing, there will be a time when diagnosing one's constitution will be done simply through physiological examination of the DNA.

1. Constitutional typing based on physical appearances

According to SCM, there are differences in the development of various regions of the body. Therefore, the particular characteristics of a constitution will manifest in the physical appearance. In most cases, the constitution can be distinguished by an accurate differentiation of the shape of the body.

For example, the TY-type persons who have Yang body types have well-developed upper bodies (the Yang region) manifesting as strong chest muscles, while their lower bodies (Yin) are weak. In contrast, the SE-type persons who have Yin body types have weaker upper bodies (Yang) and strong lower body (Yin) development manifesting as large and well-developed buttocks.

The characteristics of physical appearance in each constitution are as follows:

① The Taeyang (TY) type

The TY-type persons have well-developed upper bodies. The neck region is thick and strong and the head is large. However, the region below the waist tends to be weak. The hips are small and the leg mus-

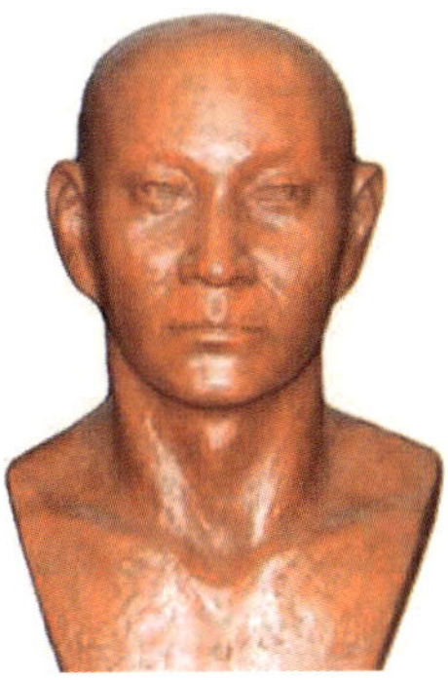

Plaster figure of the TY type

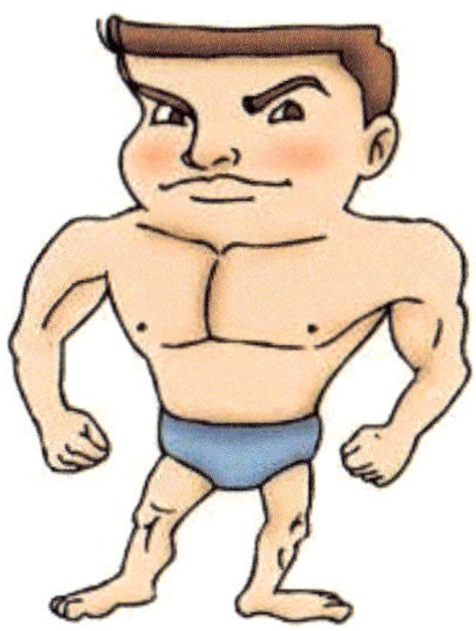

Caricature drawing of the TY type

cles are thin. Thus, in a standing position the TY-type persons seem unstable. Since the lower body is weak, TY-type persons have difficulty walking or standing for a long time. Their facial features are clearly defined and they have thin bodies.

Taeyang women, who are otherwise healthy, may have difficulty conceiving. Because they have an innate weakness in the low back and waist, their uterine development may also be weak.

On the whole, this constitution is the most difficult to recognize because it has the lowest percentage (less than 0.1% of the population) of the four constitutions.

② The Soyang (SY) type

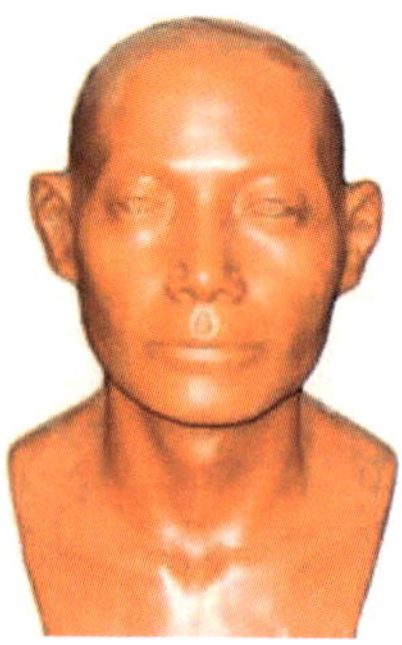

Plaster figure of the SY type

The chest and shoulder regions of the Soyang constitutions are strong and well-developed while the region below the hips is weak. On the whole, since their upper bodies are strong and their lower bodies are slight, the SY-type persons' movements are quick. Since their hip region is weak, they also appear weak in a sitting position.

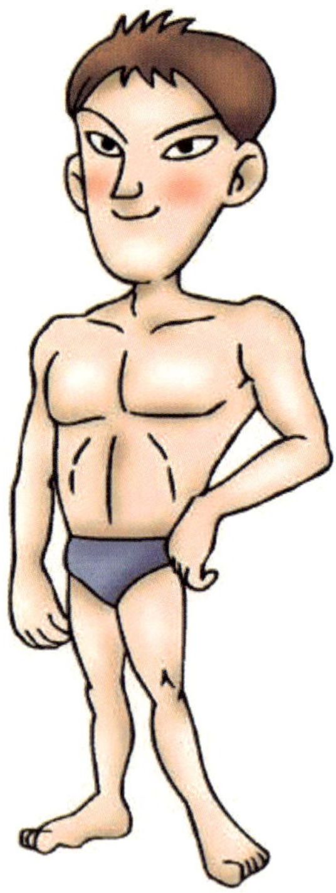

Caricature drawing of the SY type

Some SY-type persons are small in stature and have a tidy appearance, resembling the SE-type persons. It is therefore difficult at times to reach a conclusion about a constitution based solely on the physical appearance. In this case, mental characteristics and disease symptoms must be carefully observed in order to avoid misdiagnosis. There is a high proportion of the SY-type persons in the population (30%) and they are fairly easy to distinguish.

③ The Taeeum (TE) type

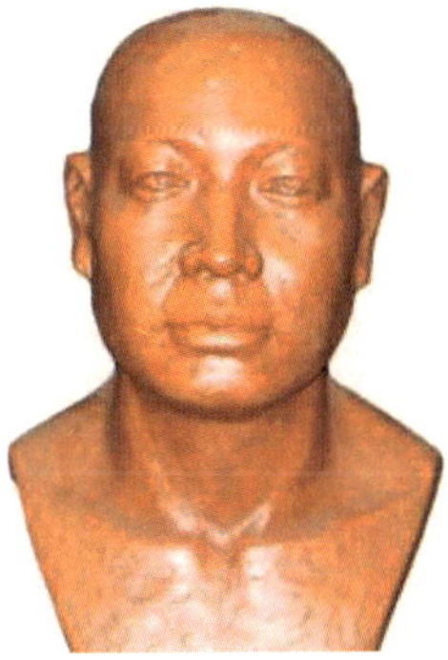

Plaster figure of the TE-type

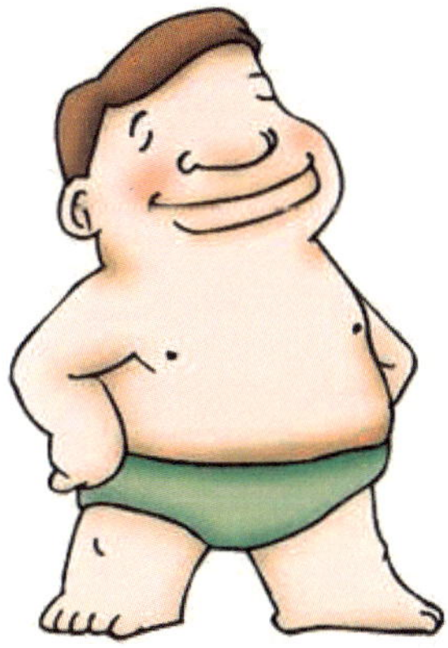

Caricature drawing of the TE-type

The Taeeum constitution has a well-developed waist region so their standing posture appears stable and strong. Their neck region, however, appears weak. The TE-type persons are normally tall and well built and rarely thin and small. Usually, the TE-type persons hold ample flesh and their physical frame is stout (strong and solid). Occasionally, a TE-type person may be thin but his or her frame will be stout nevertheless.

Even though the TE-type persons manifest clear traits, there are cases in which it is difficult to ascertain their constitution, and so it is not enough to rely solely on external appearances. In particular, since the TE-type persons' outward appearances share traits with those of

SE-type persons, caution is needed when determining their constitutions.

④ The Soeum (SE) type

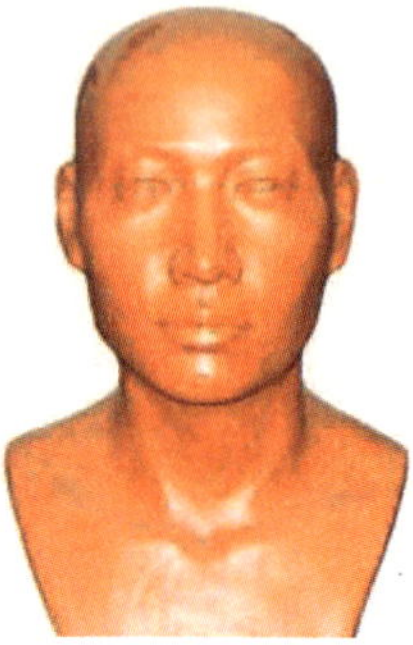

Plaster figure of the SE type

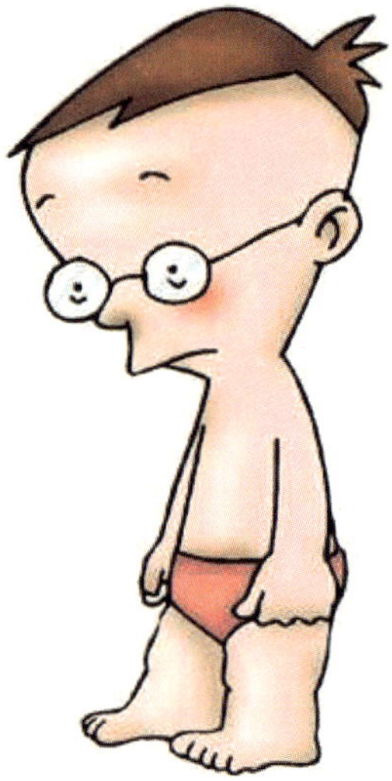

Caricature drawing of the SE type

The SE-type persons' hips and buttocks are strong and their seated posture is stable, but their chest and shoulder regions appear weak and underdeveloped. The SE-type persons are usually short in stature but at times a tall SE-type person can be found. Their lower bodies are more balanced and developed than their upper bodies. Many SE-type persons tend to walk with their bodies bent forward. Though they have stronger lower bodies compared to their upper bodies, on the whole, they have a small frame and are thin and weak.

Since female SE-type persons, in contrast to female TY-type persons, have large hips and a well-developed uterus, they can get pregnant easily and have few problems carrying a child full term.

2. Constitutional typing based on mental characteristics

Sasang constitution is characterized by its psychosomatic methodology that views the mind and body as one. The Sasang constitutional typology perceives the mind and body as inseparable, and the mental traits are intricately associated with the physical manifestations. In the same way that the physical appearances vary depending on the constitutional type, the mental characteristics also display constitutional variation. Similar to the way external appearances are expressed differently in different constitutional types, the internal mind-frame is structured differently depending on the constitutional type.

The constitution-based differences can be found in various aspects: proclivity and capacity (性質材幹: talents, natural aptitude, strengths, etc), basal tensional state of mind (恒心: the instinctive leaning of the mind when put under pressure), greed (心慾: covetous desires that surface when the mind is not adequately controlled), etc.

The differences in the initial basic mind-set give rise to the different social behaviors, such as in general aptitudes, social relationships, approaches to problem-solving, and so on. It can reasonably be assumed that observing these differences could serve as a valid and effective method of constitutional typing.

① The Taeyang (TY) constitutional type

- Proclivity and capacity -

The TY constitutional type excels at getting through to people and shows decisiveness, typically skillful at social networking. Unlike the SE type's socializing skills that are based on unassumed geniality and amiability, the TY type tend to be more actively interactive and less diffident or aloof, which together contribute to the TY type's ability of "penetration" in social relationships.

- Basal (tensional) mind-set -

A sentiment of constant urgency, or fretfulness, can be observed in the typical TY mind. This urgency needs to be kept in check in order to fare well in life. Situations tend to work out for the better when the TY person manages to control his fretfulness and ease up, whereas excessive exertion or overstraining can stir up urgency of the mind and lead to an unfortunate turn of events or cause him to lose his health.

- Personality -

Bold and active, the typical TY type tends to push onward without pulling back. A strong masculine tendency in personality is visible in the spirited manner in which they plan and conduct their affairs in life. However, many plans fall through because they overlook and neglect the importance of meticulous and detailed implementation.

- Covetous desires -

The TY mind is characterized by indiscipline (indiscretion). This attribute is accentuated when the characteristic recklessness escalates and outbalances meticulousness. One who has thus become indisciplined and heedless often knows no remorse or penitence, and this self-righteousness causes him to refuse friendly counsels, eventually leading to isolation.

As described above, the typical TY personality can either be polished into decisiveness and charisma or deteriorate into arbitrariness. The TY type persons are often clear-minded and creative, exhibiting a straightforward and great-hearted personality. They are active and enterprising and usual show decisive, assertive, and forceful ways in their behavior and comportment. They can be inattentive to details and rush on headlong, relentlessly and remorselessly. They are able to get through to people with ease, to both friends and strangers alike, but they are also easily piqued and apt to explode when faced with setbacks.

② The Soyang (SY) constitutional type

- Proclivity and capacity -

A SY type person is generally hardy and nimble, naturally gifted at conceiving and developing new ideas. He is usually venturesome and takes on new tasks with readiness and ease. Unlike those who hesitate excessively and lose the right timing or waste time mulling over past decisions, he lives by the motto "a good start is half the battle" and tackles life unhesitating and with ease. His general comportment is active and sprightly, and this natural agility confers his characteristic briskness.

- Basal (tensional) mind-set -

The typical SY type person harbors a sentiment of constant dread inside his heart. Contrary to his usual briskness in initiating new projects, he does not fare as well in tying up the loose ends. When coupled with his tendency to take on more responsibilities than he can handle and start up on new agenda before wrapping up the old ones, this can eventually lead to repeated failures in life. The fear of failing or being unable to see fruition develops into the characteristic sentiment of constant dread. Though small glitches and minor mistakes can be condoned, frequent, larger-scale problems can be demoralizing and exacerbate the inherent dread. Escalation of this sentiment can blow up into uncontrolled dread and cause the SY type person to become extremely forgetful, a sign of pathological development.

- Personality -

The generally quick-tempered SY type persons are usually quick to launch new plans but find it difficult to follow it through to the final completion. They generally lack the tenacity to persevere in face of difficulty and give up easily. They tend to juggle with many balls in the air, venturing forth too easily without necessarily following through to the end each time. They can abandon lost causes very casually and simply leave to start out on a different agenda. This can put a strain on the family, friends, or co-workers who always find themselves having to clean up somebody else's mess.

A typical SY type person enjoys the praise and glory that comes from the outside world but rarely fully appreciates the amount of energy that goes into taking care of the family. Though often quick to meddle or offer help in other people's problems, he is conversely inattentive to his own family's issues.

- Covetous desires -

The SY mind is characterized by pretentiousness, or disguising of partiality or selfishness. When the SY tendency to focus on keeping up the appearances rather than building up the solid base or improving himself is accentuated, this can lead to selfishness or partiality to those closest to himself. He can find himself basing his decisions on his mood or emotions rather than discriminating the personal and impersonal (or unimportant/trivial and important/essential) matters to make clear-cut and fair decisions. By this point, his unprincipled and temperamental behavior makes him too unreliable and haphazard to work together.

Both assertive and quick-witted, the typical SY type shows aptitude in business or social work. He can be described as generally energetic and spirited, straight-up, with a strong sense of justice and eager to serve the community. Despite the characteristic levity in behavior, the SY type person can be soft-hearted and attentive to those around him in an uncalculating way.

However, he is short-tempered and can be negligent to himself or his own family when wrapped up in the outside world. Though quick to start out on new plans, he rarely sees it through to completion because he often soon loses interest and bails out, another trait showing that perseverance is not a strong point of the SY type.

③ The Taeeum (TE) constitutional type

- Proclivity and capacity -

Owing to the steadfast and imperturbable nature, the typical TY type person usually completes the tasks he has taken on for himself. He usually finds himself settling in comfortably in any surroundings. He is a good administrator who shows perseverance and indefatigability in face of difficulties. He holds together a task with solemn dignity and sees it through to completion, rarely letting go of anything in the middle of its process.

- Basal (tensional) mind-set -

The typical TE mind always holds a sentiment of constant cowardice. He tends to resist change, which causes him to be oblivious to what is happening outside the sheltered surroundings and eventually lose self-confidence. When this cowardice is suitably controlled, he is able to function with stability both socially and at home, conveying dependability and reliability to those closest to him. However, when this innate cowardice is heightened, he can become too afraid and cautious to try and accomplish anything. This characteristic timidity can act as a stress factor and cause him to reject change and become wholly immersed in the comfortable, familiar world around him. Escalation of this sentiment can eventually evolve into unrestrained cowardice, at which point the TE-type person can experience palpitation, a sign of pathological development.

- Personality -

It is characteristic of the TE-type person to prefer inactivity, who is generally averse to change, a quality conducive to his conservative nature. He usually chooses to work within set boundaries and avoids venturing out to the competitive world outside. Once the line is drawn (around his family or his responsibility), he pays little attention to what is happening outside of his realm. And unlike the SY personality, he rarely puts his energy into the race for fame and glory that do not have real, substantial value.

- Covetous desires -

The TE mind is characterized by acquisitiveness, or avaricious pursuit of wealth. One is likely to become acquisitive when his self-preserving instincts are accentuated. Though an adequate amount of protectiveness and self-preservation could prove to be beneficial, excessive compulsion and even obsession to guard one's own possessions can lead to avariciousness.

A TE-type person has dignified features and an imposing manner of speech. He is a born moderator with natural suaveness who conveys a sense of fairness and balance. A general air of honesty and prudence can impress on those around him dependability and trustworthiness. He is conservative and resistant to change, a stickler for decorum and civility. Pertinacity and perseverance are qualities that enable his worldly accomplishments.

However, those of the TE constitutional type tend to value family matters over worldly affairs and can fall into inactivity. Behind the dignified and gentle facade, their heart often carries around suspicion and greed. They tend to avoid much activity or chattering with people, enjoying passive sports (like gambling) than strenuous exercises. They are sometimes criticized for being craven, obtuse, and slothful.

Though many heroic figures and historically important personage can be found in the TE constitutional group, a TE-type person can also be weak-willed, unsagacious, indolent, and dull-witted.

④ The Soeum (SE) constitutional type

- Proclivity and capacity -

The SE type person is usually soothing, accommodating, and calm, with a natural talent for weaving the inner fibers of an organization. His attentive, heedful, soft-spoken, and decorous qualities together attract a network of friends, and his meticulousness drives him to plan ahead of projects, preparing for all setbacks. His organizational skills are rooted in these strengths.

- Basal (tensional) mind-set -

A sentiment of constant discomfiture can be observed in the typical SE mind. Meticulousness can be interpreted as small-heartedness, and the SE type person often sweats over the small things, adept at doing commonplace work but usually the last one to try any new task that is rife with unseen possibilities. This constant feeling of disconcertion and perturbation is not only hazardous to the mentality of a person but also a debilitating influence on his physical health. Because he is so easily overwrought over trivialities, his digestion is often stalled, inducing heaviness or tightness in his stomach.

- Personality -

The SE type person's general introversion and softness can in a negative way lead to his lack of spirit or driving force. However, it they can also be the cause of the characteristic SE scrupulousness and composure. A SE type person usually makes premeditated, rational decisions and is seldom swept up emotionally at length.

- Covetous desires -

The SE mind is characterized by prevarication, or stealthy vagueness. The introversion and passivity that can be observed in the typical SE type person can sometimes cause him to be equivocal, vague, and stealthy on matters that should be clear-cut and aboveboard. His shyness and diffidence can work as an obstacle in the way of successes that could have been achieved had it been met with greater fortitude and confidence. When faced with adversity or difficulty, he shrinks back to his corner rather than rise to the challenge, refusing to venture out further into the seemingly hostile world. This detached, withdrawn evasiveness is in fact vague prevarication, the covetous desire found in the SE mind.

A typical SE type person's comportment, manner of speech, and features are generally unpretentious, unassumed, dainty, and deft. He usually has a compliant, placating, calm, and friendly personality. He shows keen judgment, meticulousness planning, and organized thought processes.

However, he rarely voices his opinions actively, discouraged by his own introversion and shyness. His soft-hearted and diffident nature effectively drowns out potential forcefulness and ambitious drive. Those of the SE constitutional type can exhibit strong individualist or egoist tendencies, responding vehemently to outside interference, the ones to calculate every gain and loss. They are predisposed to jealousy and envy, also notorious for carrying around old grudges for years on end.

The general mental characteristics described above could aid the constitutional typing process in those who exhibit strong constitutional tendencies, but mental attributes can show great variation depending on many factors, such as his educational background or life experiences, that can either accentuate or muffle certain personality traits.

It is dangerous to believe that certain mental characteristics are seen exclusively in specific constitutional types. For instance, urgency or discomfiture could be seen outside of the TY or SE types, respectively, because they are common emotional manifestations that can be relatively more visible in some and less so in others. The Four

Beginnings (or Sprouts) of the mind, namely compassion (giving rise to benevolence), shame/dislike (giving rise to righteousness), modesty/deference (giving rise to respect/courtesy), and distinguishing right from wrong (giving rise to wisdom), that were proposed by Mencius can be seen in all of the four constitutional types; however, the balance between the most accentuated Beginning and the least accentuated Beginning and the way they interweave and interact are different in each constitutional type, which causes the constitutional variations in mental characteristics.

3. Constitutional typing based on pathological patterns

In general, traditional eastern medicine does not associate any one particular disease pattern with any given constitution. In other words, there is no consideration given to the reasons behind why some people are afflicted with certain diseases while others are not. Traditional eastern medicine views the human body as an innately harmonized and balanced entity. Diseases arise due to certain factors inside or outside of the body that break that balance. Therefore, eastern medicine differentiates the unbalanced state into excesses and deficiencies. The treatment principle focuses on restoring balance by eliminating these disruptive factors.

In contrast, SCM views the human body as an inherently incomplete and unbalanced system. Harmony does not arise automatically but can only be obtained by conscious effort. There are imperfections and imbalances not only in the body, but also in the mind. No one is born a sage. It is the basic view of SCM that although one may be born with an unbalanced mind, by cultivating one's mind it is possible to become a sage. Since the body is also not innately balanced, health can only be obtained by controlling one's physical imbalances. Although external factors do, in fact, cause diseases, they do not bring about illness until they affect the internal body. From this perspective, intrinsic factors are considered to be the root cause of diseases.

One symptom can represent either a disease state or a healthy condition depending upon a person's constitution. In addition, each constitution exhibits particular signs of disease as well as particular disease progressions. For example, spontaneous sweating is a healthy sign for TE-type persons but is unhealthy for the SE-type persons. There are also certain diseases that only afflict particular constitutions. In other words, there exist constitutional syndromes. Once these factors are recognized, a natural and effective treatment method can be instituted. Inversely, constitutions can be differentiated through the particular characteristics of diseases.

The state of health, aptly called the "healthy state," varies across each constitution. For instance, ease in urination is the healthy state for TY-type, while sound digestion is the healthy state of the SE-type persons. In the same way, the signs of disease vary according to each constitution. An initial or mild imbalance is known as a "mild disease" and is viewed not only to contrast a healthy state, but also to contrast a "severe disease," which indicates that the disease is either critical or extremely difficult to treat.

In such a way, there are differing states of health and constitutional syndromes, as well as, differing progression of disease in each constitution. Therefore, the constitution can be identified by careful examination of these factors.

① The Taeyang (TY) type

Healthy State

TY-type persons are in a healthy state if they urinate a large amount without any difficulty. One way to differentiate a TY-type person is that he or she will have ease in urination when healthy but will have discomfort when not feeling well.

Mild Disease

TY-type persons have a mild disease if they have a great deal of saliva or foam in their mouths. This needs immediate treatment.

Severe Disease

Yul Gyuk or dysphagia is the constitutional disease of the TY-type persons. When this disease worsens, the person will find it difficult to swallow food. Even if he or she is able to swallow the food, it will not descend to the stomach, but instead will be vomited up immediately. At this time, the person can feel a cool wind blowing in the esophagus. These symptoms will distinguish a TY-type person and are considered critical symptoms.

Yul Gyuk (dysphagia), Ban Wyi (vomiting) and Hae Yuk (lower body weakness) are all important symptoms in differentiating the TY constitutional type but they do not appear until the situation is serious. Thus TY-type persons generally appear to be healthy. Ban Wyi appears as epigastric bloating and fullness after eating with vomiting afterwards. Hae Yuk appears as fatigue of the whole body that results in lethargy, weakness of the legs, thinning of the body, and no desire to talk. At times, Yul Gyuk can occur in an elderly SE-type person, so they must not be misdiagnosed as TY-type persons.

When a person exhibits the above-mentioned constitutional syndromes and disease progression, the person can be discerned as a TY-type person.

② The Soyang (SY) type

Healthy State

For the SY-type, good bowel movements indicate a healthy state. When the healthy bowel movements turn into constipation as the body becomes ill, the person can be considered to be of the SY-type.

The TE-type persons are highly susceptible to constipation. However, it is generally not considered a disease state. In contrast, the SY-type persons are healthy when they have good bowel movements, and unhealthy when they have constipation. Thus, constipation is a clear indication of a disease in the SY-type.

Mild Disease

Constipation indicates a mild disease. If a SY-type person has constipation, it should be considered to be an unhealthy condition and a treatment plan should be devised immediately. Disease progression in the SY-type person is quick and so constipation should not be taken lightly.

Severe Disease

When the SY-type person has constipation for two or three consecutive days with heat and a stifling sensation in the chest, he or she has a severe disease. In contrast to the SE-type who experiences ice cold abdomens with continuous diarrhea, the SY-type will develop a heat sensation in the chest when the constipation continues.

The Soyang constitution can be differentiated by disease symptoms once a person understands the healthy state and the progression of a disease.

③ The Taeeum (TE) type

Healthy State

The TE-type persons are in a healthy state if they sweat frequently. If a person sweats easily even though they only move slightly or if they sweat profusely during the wintertime after eating warm foods, they are of the TE constitutional type. In contrast to the SE-type persons who would feel sick and exhausted after sweating profusely, the TE-type persons do not feel even the slightest discomfort; they may actually feel refreshed. A person who sweats in large quantities when there is no disease present has a high probability of being a TE-type person.

Mild Disease

For the TE-type persons, having firm skin and an inability to sweat indicates a disease state. If there is an absence of sweating, other symptoms will soon follow and the disease will worsen. A person in this state should, therefore, be treated immediately.

Severe Disease

If the small intestine (situated in the Lower Middle Burner) feels blocked as though a fog is clogging up that region, then the disease is considered to be severe.

Usually, profuse sweating is a sign of deficiency or disease. However, in the case of the TE-type persons, it is a sign of health. The ideal sweat beads of a TE-type person are thick and stay on the skin for a long time.

An understanding of this information about health and disease states should allow for the differentiation of the TE constitutional type.

④ The Soeum (SE) type

Healthy State

The SE-type persons feel healthy when their digestion is good. They generally have weak Spleen Qi, and so once the Spleen Qi is revived and digestion is improved, they are in a healthy state. If the SE-type persons have no appetite and develop fullness in the chest after eating, they will feel bodily discomfort.

Mild Disease

Profuse sweating indicates a mild disease. Unlike the TE-type persons, spontaneous sweating in the SE-type persons indicates that a disease has already progressed and it must be treated quickly.

Severe Disease

A SE-type person with continuous diarrhea and a cold abdomen has a severe disease. This constitution has a weak Spleen and Stomach and so they tend to develop many diseases associated with that weakness. People with chronic digestive problems are usually SE-type and although they may manifest other diseases, these diseases are not of great concern as long as the digestive system is healthy. No matter the disease, as long as there is no excessive sweating and no problem drinking water, it is not considered to be a serious disease.

Once this information about healthy and disease states is understood, the Soeum constitution can be differentiated.

Clinical Applications of Sasang Constitutional Medicine

1. Constitution differentiation

While there are many different methods for classifying Sasang types, the three most important aspects are appearance, mind/nature (心性), and illness.

Appearance refers to body type and facial appearance. This includes simple observations of the face and its' overall configuration, as well as the atmosphere that can be detected based on the movements and speech patterns. Each type has a set of distinct physical traits, which may provide clues for differentiation. Although the overall size of the body is subject to change, the frame does not. However, observing body type and appearance alone does not provide enough information to differentiate the constitutions.

Mind/nature is reflected in one's personality (性質), capacity (ability to take care of matters), determination (恒心; thoughts that one carries in their hearts), and covetous desires (心慾). There are very distinct personality features for each type, and these features are very important. However, these features cannot be used as the primary evaluation tool, as there are individuals who do not show their true personalities. In these cases, the patient is put in an urgent situation to examine their true intentions.

Differentiation based on illness is possible based on healthful states and symptoms that are displayed when one is not feeling well; these states and symptoms are significantly different for each Sasang type. However, some Sasang types only display symptoms when conditions are severe. Therefore, Sasang differentiation that is based on illness alone is not a complete method.

For accurate differentiation, it is recommended that all three aspects, appearance, mind/nature, and illness, are reviewed before reaching a conclusion.

1) Sasang type differentiations based on appearance

① Taeyangin

In appearance, Taeyangin have large upper chests, thick necks, and large heads, which are all areas that pertain to the lungs (肺). They have an overall image that makes them appear as though the qi is surging upwards. As such, Taeyangin resemble 'lions'; however, they are weak below the waist in areas that pertain to the liver (肝). They have small, lean legs, and they may appear unstable when standing. Taeyangin tend to have very prominent facial features and rarely become overweight. Taeyangin are the least common of the four Sasang types and are difficult to find.

② Soyangin

Soyangin have a large chest, which is related to the spleen (脾). They have very broad shoulders that result in an 'eagle'-like appearance. In contrast, the kidneys (腎), which relate to the rear, are very small, which results in an unstable appearance when sitting. Many Soyangin have small, round heads that protrude anteriorly and posteriorly. Their eyes look sharp, and the mouth is small with thin lips. The chin tends to be pointy, and the skin is fair yet dry. Soyangin do not perspire, and they have clear and high-pitched voices. They do not give much thought to what they say. Soyangin may appear hasty because their speech and movements are abrupt.

③ Taeeumin

The low back area is strong, which gives Taeeumin a stout and stable posture when standing. However, they have a relatively thin neck. Many Taeeumin have a very large frame. Their hands and feet are large in size and easily become dry and chapped during the winter. They are often sweaty, and even the smallest movements may cause them to perspire. Taeeumin tend to have prominent facial features.

They have a stable gait, but their upper torso gravitates anteriorly as they walk. Taeyangins' waist and abdominal areas appear to be oversized, and they may look arrogant.

④ Soeumin

The buttocks are developed, which provides stability in the sitting position. However, they have small chests that make them appear as though they are hunched forward. They usually have stronger lower than upper bodies. When they walk, they hunch forward and flop their bodies. Because Soeumin tend to have a stronger lower body compared to their upper body, they look petite, thin, and often weak. Their facial features are not prominent but are harmonious. Soeumin appear modest, and have petite facial features. Their skin is soft, and perspiration is sparse. They tend to smile with their eyes during conversations.

2) Constitution determinations based on mind and nature

Mind and nature refer to proclivity and capacity (性質材幹: talent, special abilities, and strengths), covetous determination (恒心: thoughts that are always in their hearts), and desires (心慾: greed that surfaces when mind and nature are not properly controlled).

① Taeyangin

Taeyangin are very talented at socializing. They are not intimidated by the presence of others and are very active. They make friends very easily. Taeyangin tend to only move forward, and do not move backwards (慾進而不慾退). They rarely look at their surroundings and only face forward. They may develop an urgent mind (急迫之心: a state of being hasty). When mind and nature are not controlled, they develop self-indulgence (放縱之心) and become self-righteous or arrogant.

② Soyangin

Soyangin are active and swift in their movements. They are outspoken and are good at generating and pursuing ideas. However, they do not often see matters through to their conclusion (慾擧而不慾措). They tend to focus more on matters outside the home and neglect what occurs inside (the mind and the home). This results in an anxious mind (懼心). When Soyangin are confronted with serious problems, anxiety may develop into fear, which may in turn cause memory impairments. This is a dangerous state.

When they only focus on matters outside the home and neglect matters inside the home, they may develop an irrational mind (偏私之心: the tendency to only focus on personal things).

③ Taeeumin

Taeeumin are calm and determined. They successfully complete things that they have started or have been assigned. However, because they prefer to remain still without moving (慾靜而不慾動), they are aware of their minds and homes, but do not know much about the outside world. This causes a cowardly mind (怯心: the tendency to be careful). When this anxiety becomes severe, they may develop palpitations (怔忡).

When the tendency to protect the inside becomes too strong, they may develop a materialistic mind (物慾之心). It is good to focus on personal achievements and protect personal possessions, but when this tendency becomes too strong and love becomes an obsession, greed can develop.

④ Soeumin

Soeumin are gentle, calm and meticulous. They are detail oriented, and precisely plan matters to attract other people's minds. However, they always prefer to stay in without coming forth (慾處而不慾出). In other words, they are more introverted than extroverted. They are not very ambitious. Because they have such introverted characteristics, they can be quite anxious (不安定之心). Soeumin have a tendency to be anxious all the time.

When these traits of Soeumin become too strong, they may become complacent. Even in matters that can bring great success, they are reluctant to try new things because of their introverted nature. When they face hardships, rather than trying to overcome difficulties, Soeumin tend to sit back and wait. This complacent nature is be a negative characteristic(偸逸之心) of the Soeumin type .

3) Constitution differentiations that are based on illness (病證)

Each Sasang constitution is susceptible to a distinct set of illnesses. These illnesses are called 'constitutional illnesses' (體質病證) and are caused by a lack of control of daily habits. There are very distinct definitions of health (完實無病), unhealthy states (大病), and severe diseases (重病) for each Sasang type.

A healthful condition refers to the state of health that is unique to each Sasang type. Unhealthy states are not serious illnesses but are transitory phases between health and pathology. Severe disease refers to a condition in which the person is at his/her weakest.

① Taeyangin

Taeyangin are healthy when they urinate well and have clear urine. When there is saliva or foam reflux in the mouth, they are in an unhealthy state. When the body is not adequately nurtured, more severe conditions may develop. Regurgitation (噎膈證) can occur when Taeyangin cannot swallow food, or when they swallow food that does not successfully reach the stomach. When this occurs, the entire body feels heavy and the legs feel weak, and the patient does not want to move or speak, which is called paraparesis (解㑊證). Both regurgitation (噎膈證) and paraparesis (解㑊) are severe conditions in which there is an upsurge (逆上) in qi, which causes deficiencies in the lower body and excess in the upper body (下虛上實). These are Taeyangin's illnesses.

② Soyangin

Soyangin are healthy when they adequately defecate. When a person adequately defecates but becomes constipated when unwell, it is likely that they are Soyangin. If constipation is observed in a Soyangin, they are in an unhealthy state that may develop into more serious problems. If a Soyangin feels stuffy in the chest and is unable to defecate for 2-3 days, they may have a severe disease. Soyangin's illnesses are internal heat (內熱) due to fire (火) and heat (熱).

③ Taeeumin

Taeeumin are healthy when they adequately perspire. When the skin is so dense and tight (稠密) that it interferes with proper perspiration, they are in a state of severe disease that may cause further problems. When Taeeumin have diarrhea and feel heavy and full in the lower abdomen, they may have a severe disease. Tidal fevers (燥熱病證) that are due to improper perspiration, urination, and defecation are a state of illness that are observed in Taeeumin.

④ Soeumin

Soeumin are considered healthy if they can properly digest food. When they are not able properly digest food or when they excessively perspire, they are in an unhealthy state. When diarrhea does not stop and the lower abdomen feels cold, they are in a state of severe illness.

Soeumin illnesses can be divided into two conditions, the cold stomach syndrome (胃寒病證), which is a condition of coldness in the digestive system, or the yang deficiency syndrome (陽虛病證), which is due to excessive sweating.

2. Constitutional Illnesses

1) Illnesses that are prevalent in Taeyangin

Taeyangin have a strong tendency to expel energy outwards due to their large (strong) lungs, but they lack the ability to take qi inward, due to a small (weak) liver. The upper body is large, which pertains to the lungs, while the lower body is smaller. The neck is especially thick and strong. Taeyangin have a large head but a weak lower body with small buttocks and thin legs. They appear somewhat unstable in a standing position. Taeyangin find it hard to stand or walk for long periods of time.

In their structure and function, Taeyangin have a tendency to upsurge and expel but lack an ability to accumulate. This may cause illness. Illnesses that are commonly found in Taeyangin are paraparesis (解㑊) and regurgitation (噎膈).

Paraparesis (解㑊) is a condition in which an excessive upsurge of qi has led to excess in the upper areas and deficiencies in the lower areas (上盛下虛). The legs are weak. There is no swelling, pain (腫痛), or numbness, but the legs do not receive the qi that is needed to walk properly.

Regurgitation (噎膈) is a condition in which energy is expelled outwards, but less energy is consumed by the middle and lower energies. When food passes through the esophagus to enter the stomach, there is a sense of obstruction or actual vomiting.

To treat this condition, it is important to eliminate qi upsurges in the upper body (上體). To achieve this goal, it is important not to become angry. Before prescribing medication, it is important to find peace of mind, stay away from anger, remain calm, and avoid greasy foods.

2) Illnesses that are prevalent in Soyangin

Soyangin have a weak urogenital system and therefore often have bladder or kidney disease. Soyangin may have edema due to dysfunctions in urination.

When Soyangin illnesses are mostly hot (熱性) in nature, they lack the yin qi that can yield an excess of heat and fire and causes heat-type diseases. Types of diseases that are prevalent in Soyangin are edema due to insufficient urination and heat patterns in the chest that are accompanied by constipation. When the chest heat pattern remains unresolved for an extended period of time, it becomes a chronic condition that is called yin deficiency afternoon heat syndrome.

Soyangin illnesses can either be of an excessive heat (實熱) or a deficient heat (虛熱) type. The excessive heat-type syndrome is the Hyunggyeok-yeol symptomatic pattern (胸膈熱證). In this syndrome, an inability to defecate causes fire heat (火熱) to upsurge. Symptoms include a red face, an increase in thirst, vexation in the chest, and insomnia. Diabetes yang toxin skin spots (skin rashes with itchiness) can develop when Soyangin are prescribed heat-type medications that are contraindicated. Children may develop convulsions. Parts of the head that are affected include the eyes, nose, ears, lips, teeth, larynx, and other parts, which become inflammatory and bloodshot. In these cases, constipation aggravates the condition. Herbal medicine can clear the heat inside, treat constipation, clear the urine, resolve thirst, and clear the vexing heat in the chest.

When these symptoms are not properly treated, a Eumheo-oyeol symptomatic pattern (陰虛午熱證) develops.

This is a state of repeated episodes of tidal fevers (潮熱) in the afternoon. These result from heat that is produced under deficient circumstances. This is a state of yin deficiency and yang exuberance, which occurs when the Soyangin have lost control of their lifestyle and have not appropriately treated their illnesses. In this case, it is important to replenish yin (補陰) to compensate for constitutional shortcomings.

3) Illnesses that are prevalent in Taeeumin

Taeeumin are subtyped into two categories for discussing illnesses: cold-type Taeeumin and heat-type Taeeumin.

Cold-type Taeeumin are very similar to Soeumin. They are sensitive to cold climates and easily catch cold. They frequently have diarrhea. In contrast, heat-type Taeeumin easily develop constipation, obesity, thirst, and irritation in the chest. By observing their usual conditions, it is possible to differentiate between cold-type and heat-type Taeeumin. Heat types often present with problems in the circulatory system due to constipation and obesity. Cold-type Taeeumin perspire well and thus may not have circulatory issues but may suffer from frequent diarrhea and/or common colds.

Taeeumin can easily become obese. For children, sibling rivalry or peer pressure may cause anxiety. As a way to address these issues, Taeeumin develop a strong appetite because they are not confident about their activities outside the home. They do not like to socialize and prefer to stay at home. They do not like to move and avoid exercise. Constipation and obesity are common in Taeeumin.

For adults, an undisciplined diet and a lack of exercise may cause obesity, circulatory problems, diabetes, and stroke, which are prevalent conditions in Taeeumin. Additionally, nervousness due to accumulating stress may cause arteriosclerosis, hypertension, cardiovascular diseases, diabetes, and stroke. Obesity and constipation may interfere with proper digestion and cause an accumulation in phlegm (痰飮) (abnormally accumulated bodily fluid), which in turn can cause arthritis, allergies, psychological problems, and skin problems.

Taeeumin should be aware of the following recommendations.

First, it is possible to enhance circulation by sweating through proper exercise and bathing. Taeeumin are healthy when they adequately perspire. Soeumin are healthy when they do not sweat, but Taeeumin are ill when they do not sweat.

Second, to aid in proper digestion, Taeeumin must maintain a healthy weight and eat meals with sufficient amounts of fiber-rich foods to ensure proper defecation.

Third, emotional anxiety and stress should be minimized. Actively participating in experiences outside of the home can help the inner self relate to the external world. These experiences help broaden Taeeumin's perceptions, purify their mind and nature and contribute to improvements in their constitution.

4) Illnesses that are prevalent in Soeumin

Soeumin have large kidneys and small spleens (腎大脾小). Because the spleen and stomach (脾胃) are small (小; weak), Soeumin have gastrointestinal problems.

They cannot digest foods as well as others types, even when they do not eat much. They have pain under the sternum, feel uneasy and stuffy in the abdominal region, and have trouble digesting food. In Soeumin, the end of the sternum feels painful, the stomach feels bloated, there are frequent complaints of stomach pain, and they have diarrhea after eating cold foods or drinking beer. This type of diarrhea is not due to intestinal problems but manifests from problems in the stomach. Because they are born with a weak and cold digestive system, they cannot properly digest food. Exposure to cold foods may trigger diarrhea. Therefore, dyspepsia, gastritis, gastroptosis, habitual abdominal pain, and other acute/chronic illnesses of the gastrointestinal system are common conditions in Soeumin.

Soeumin do not have a large body mass, and their body is cold. Therefore, they should not sweat. Sweating will cause deficiencies in qi, thereby causing the body to become frail. When Soeumin habitually sweat, it is a sign that they are not well. In contrast, Taeeumin tend to have a very large body. They should frequently perspire to ensure proper circulation. However, Soeumin are the opposite because they are well when their skin is tight and they do not perspire. When Soeumin become very tired or participate in aggressive sporting activities, they may sweat too much, lose their qi, become cold and develop illnesses.

Soeumin have a weak digestive system, which may lead to several problems. Even when there are other symptoms, when there are no gastrointestinal symptoms, there are no serious problems. Soeumin are timid and introverted. They can easily become anxious about the smallest things, which may cause dyspepsia or neurosis and insomnia. Therefore, anxiety should be controlled, and Soeumin should attempt to be more adventurous to prevent psychological problems. Soeumin are weak and frail. Because their bodies are cold, they should refrain from participating in aggressive sporting activities or being overworked. Soeumin must keep the body warm at all times and avoid overeating and cold foods to maintain a healthy state in the gastrointestinal system.

3. Acupuncture based on Sasang constitutions

1) Taekuk acupuncture method (太極鍼法)

Constitution	鑑別穴 (Replenish)	治療穴 Tonify	治療穴 Sedate	病別 治療穴	
Taeyangin	少府(火) (HT 8)	太衝 (LR 3)	太淵 (LU 9)	Lungs>Spleen>Kidneys>Liver. Spleen, Lungs=Drain Kidneys, Liver=Replenish	Lungs-太淵 Spleen-太白 Liver-太衝 Kidneys-太谿
Taeeumin	靈道(金) (HT 4)	太淵 (LU 9)	太衝 (LR 3)	Liver>Kidneys>Spleen>Lungs. Kidneys, Liver=Drain Lungs, Spleen=Replenish	
Soyangin	少海(水) (HT 3)	太谿 (KI 3)	太白 (SP 3)	Spleen>Lungs>Liver>Kidneys. Spleen, Lungs=Drain Liver, Kidneys=Replenish	
Soeumin	神門(土) (HT 7)	太白 (SP 3)	合谷 (LI 4)	Kidneys>Liver>Lungs>Spleen. Kidneys, Liver=Drain Lungs, Spleen=Replenish	

2) Acupuncture based on constitution (體質針法)

Fundamental Formulas of 8 Constitutions					
Name of constitutions	Symbol of formula / Therapeutical process		Name of constitutions	Symbol of formula / Therapeutical process	
Hespero	I AC	I'7c IX'9p I'9p	Hespera	VIII RP	X'10c VIII'10c IV'4p VIII'4p
Saturno	IX AM	V'5c IX'5 VII'7p IX'7p	Saturna	VI RP	VI'8c II'2p VI'2p
Jupito	I RC	VIII'7p I'7p III'3c I'3c	Jupita	VIII AP	VI'6p VIII'6p IV'4c VIII'4c
Mercurio	IX RM	V'5p IX'5p I'1c IX'1c	Mercuria	VI AP	IV'4p VI'4p II'2c VI'2c

Legend:

Symbols of ZANG system
I. Liver
III. Heart
V. Pancreas
VI.I Lung
IX. Kidney
III. Simpo (Pericardium)

Symbols of FU system
II. Gall bladder
IV. Small intestine
VI. Stomach
VIII. Large intestine
X. Urinary bladder
IV. Samcho (Triple warmer)

체질	치료방법				체질	치료방법			
	補		瀉			補		瀉	
I A-담허체질 (담정격)	UB66 (통곡)	GB43 (협계)	LI1 (상양)	GB44 (규음)	IR-담실체질 (담승격)	LI1 (상양)	GB44 (규음)	SI5 (양곡)	GB38 (양보)
II A-간허체질 (간정격)	K10 (음곡)	LIV8 (곡천)	L8 (경거)	LIV4 (중봉)	IIR-간실체질 (간승격)	L8 (경거)	LIV8 (중봉)	H8 (소부)	LIV2 (행간)
III A-소장허체질 (소장정격)	GB41 (임읍)	SI3 (후계)	UB66 (통곡)	SI2 (전곡)	III R-소장실체질 (소장승격)	UB66 (통곡)	SI2 (상양)	ST36 (삼리)	SI8 (임읍)
III A-삼초허체질 (삼초정격)	GB41 (임읍)	T3 (중저)	UB66 (통곡)	T2 (액문)	III R-삼초실체질 (삼초승격)	UB66 (통곡)	T2 (액문)	ST36 (삼리)	T10 (천정)
IV A-심허체질 (심정격)	LIV1 (대돈)	H9 (소충)	K10 (음곡)	H3 (소해)	IV R-심실체질 (심승격)	K10 (곡택)	H3 (소해)	SP3 (태백)	H7 (신문)
IV A-심포허체질 (심포정격)	LIV1 (대돈)	P9 (중충)	K10 (음곡)	P3 (곡택)	IV R-심포실체질 (심포승격)	K10 (곡택)	P3 (곡택)	SP3 (태백)	P7 (대릉)
V A-위허체질 (위정격)	SI5 (양곡)	ST41 (해계)	GB41 (임읍)	ST43 (함곡)	VR-위실체질 (위승격)	GB41 (임읍)	ST43 (양곡)	LI1 (상양)	ST45 (여태)
VI A-비허체질 (비정격)	H8 (소부)	SP2 (대도)	LIV1 (대돈)	SP1 (은백)	VI R-비실체질 (비승격)	LIV1 (은백)	SP1 (대돈)	L8 (경거)	SP5 (상구)
VII A-대허체질 (대장정격)	ST36 (삼리)	LI11 (곡지)	SI5 (양곡)	LI5 (양계)	VII R-대장실체질 (대장승격)	SI5 (양곡)	LI5 (양계)	UB66 (통곡)	LI2 (이간)
VIII A-폐허체질 (폐정격)	SP3 (태백)	L9 (태간)	H8 (소부)	L10 (어제)	VIII R-폐실체질 (폐승격)	H8 (소부)	L10 (어제)	K10 (음곡)	L5 (척택)
XI A-방광허체질 (방광정격)	LI1 (상양)	UB67 (지음)	ST36 (삼리)	UB54 (위중)	XI R-방광실체질 (방광승격)	ST36 (삼리)	UB54 (위중)	GB41 (임읍)	UB65 (속골)
X A-신허체질 (신정격)	L8 (경거)	K7 (부류)	SP3 (태백)	K3 (태계)	XR-신실체질 (신승격)	SP3 (태백)	K3 (태계)	LIV1 (대돈)	K1 (용천)

24 Constitutions: the root of the disease replenishes and eliminates the origin and then the symptom
二十四體質 病根補瀉原則表

4. Managing each Sasang type

Dr. Je-Ma Lee (李濟馬) introduced management plans for each Sasang type in addition to treatment with herbal medicines. The plans include management of the mind and body (心身), diet, and social life.

1) Mind and body (心身) management

In Sasang medicine, people are perceived as spiritually and physically (心身) inadequate at birth. Such incompleteness cannot be naturally resolved. A state of balance can only be acquired through effort. Although external pathogens may directly cause a specific illness, internal self-regulation can help heal or prevent illness before it causes problems. Therefore, nurturing the mind and body is based on the theory that controlling the mind can help control qi and thereby prevent illness. Careful observation of one's general well-being can help maintain a heathy state in the body.

① Taeyangin

In Taeyangin, qi can easily rise upwards. Therefore, they should take care not to become angry, as this will cause an upsurge in qi. They should always try to control their irrational habits. They should also be careful to not become aggressive.

It is important to examine the amount of urination. Foam or saliva that frequently well up in the mouth or hard tender points that form at the tip of the sternum are signs of unhealthiness. When Taeyangin feel weakness in the legs or cannot swallow food, patients should be treated immediately as this condition is fatal.

② Taeeumin

In Taeeumin, qi can quite easily move downwards. Taeeumin should take care to not be overjoyed, as joy will make the qi sink inwards. They should also attempt to take an interest in the outside world and try to become more adventurous.

Taeeumin are healthy when they adequately perspire. When they do not or when they only perspire in certain areas, such as the upper back or neck without sweat on the face or soles/palms, they are unhealthy.

③ Soyangin

Soyangin are emotionally sensitive, tend to easily develop heat and should be careful not to become excessively sad. Additionally, it is important to refrain from overestimating oneself and belittling others. In addition, they should take more interest in matters inside the home than matters outside the home. Soyangin should not have unresolved duties.

Soyangin are only healthy when they regularly defecate every day. When they do not, they will feel uncomfortable and stuffy in the chest.

When Soyangin present with constipation or a headache, use caution. When they present with even a small amount of nasal bleeding, it should be viewed as a state of vomiting blood. When cool saliva is secreted in the mouth, it should be treated as vomiting, even when there is no actual vomit. Stroke and edema may progress quite quickly in Soyangin. These conditions should be treated immediately.

④ Soeumin

It is important that Soeumin take precaution to not be overly happy, as it may cause the qi to sink downwards. They should try to be one step ahead and more adventurous, without settling. Anxiety and jealousy should also be kept under control.

Soeumin should be able to adequately digest their food, and heavy perspiration is not a good sign. A fever that is accompanied by heavy sweating and continuous diarrhea with a very cold sensation in the lower abdomen is a critical condition.

2) Nutrition for each Sasang type

In Korean medicine, food is as important as medicinal herbs. This concept is described by the famous phrase 'medicine and food share origins (醫食同源).' Food, in Korean medicine, is not perceived as nutrients and calories, but as qi and substances with characteristics that trigger changes in the body.

Because foods are often more neutral than medicinal herbs, it is difficult to recognize harms that can be inflicted by foods in a healthy state. However, in an unhealthy state, when the immune system and resistance to disease is low, food has a larger effect on the body.

In Sasang medicine, the four Sasang types are very distinct in nature (性品) and visceral (臟器) characteristics. Therefore, qi (氣運) is biased in a certain direction. In Taeyangin (太陽人) and Soyangin (少陽人), qi is biased upwards and outwards, while in Soeumin (少陰人) and Taeumin (太陰人), qi is biased downwards and inwards. In a healthy state, the human body can regulate such imbalances. However, states of emotional distress or irregular habits and diets disrupt the harmony of the qi and cause illnesses. A full understanding of the nature and visceral characteristics for each Sasang type, knowledge of qi and the flavors of foods can help a practitioner plan an appropriate diet for each Sasang type.

① Taeyangin

Qi in Taeyangin tends to surge upwards. It is recommended that they consume foods that have pure qi and/or a bland taste that are easily digested and absorbed, such as seafood, which has a low fat content, or vegetables. These help the qi flow downwards.

Beneficial foods	Fagopyrum esculentum, Vitis coignetiae , gooseberry, grapes, persimmon, cherry ,quince, Brasenia schreber pine pollen, sea cucumber, carp, clams, crab, etc
Harmful foods	spicy foods that are heavily spiced or foods that are greasy
Recommended herbs	Acanthopanacis Cortex, quince , gooseberry , pine needles, goldfish, etc

② Taeeumin

Taeeumin are quite large and have good gastrointestinal functioning. They have a tendency to overeat, and obesity, hypertension, and constipation are common problems for Taeeumin. They should avoid spicy foods or foods that are rich in fat and refrain from overeating.

Beneficial foods	wheat, beans, sweet potato, pearl barley, corn, peanut, unpolished rice, beef, milk and diary products, chestnut, pine nut, walnut, gingko, white radish, bellflower roots, carrot, deodeok, bracken, seaweed, dried seaweed, yam, etc
Harmful foods	chicken, dog meat, pork, garlic, ginger, pepper, honey, ginseng, coffee, etc
Recommended herbs	Dioscoreae Rhizoma, Schisandrae Fructus, Puerariae Radix, Cervi Parvum Cornu, Ursi Fel, Moschus, Liriopis Tuber

③ Soyangin

Soyangin have heat in their digestive systems and are impulsive. They should consume many cold foods, vegetables, and seafood to help remove the heat and restore peace of mind.

Beneficial foods	barley, red bean, mung beans, cabbage, cucumber, lettuce, burdock, pumpkin, eggplant, watermelon, oriental melon, strawberries, banana, Welsh onion, pineapple, oyster, sea cucumber, sea squirt, abalones, shrimp, lobster, carp, pork, beer, iced products, etc
Harmful foods	Welsh onion, garlic, pepper, ginger, pepper, chicken, dog meat, deer meat, goat meat, honey, ginseng, etc
Recommended herbs	Rehmanniae Radix Preparata, Corni Fructus, Lycii Fructus, Rehmanniae Radix Crudus

④ Soeumin

Soeumin have a weak digestive system and must eat small portions at a time. They should always remember to eat foods that have warm properties or are slightly spiced. Greasy or cold foods may adversely affect the digestive system and cause diarrhea and dyspepsia.

Beneficial foods	glutinous rice, potatoes, honey, chicken, dog meat, deer meat, goat meat, sheep milk, pollack, sea bream, croaker, anchovy, croaker, apples, tomatoes, peaches, jujubes, spinach, Welsh onion, garlic, ginger, pepper, mustard, etc
Harmful foods	cold noodles, oriental melon, watermelon, cold milk, ice products, beer, barley rice, pork, flour, etc
Recommended herbs	ginseng, Eleocharitis Dulcis Rhizoma, Astragali Radix, Angelica Gigantis Radix, Cnidii Rhizoma, Cinnamomi Cortex

Food that is suitable for each type should be understood as a way to help the body return to a balanced state. Eating only one or two foods that are thought to be beneficial for each constitutional type for an extended period of time can impact ones health.

3) Social life management for each Sasang type

① Taeyangin

Taeyangin are very active and adventurous. They are social and easily make new friends. However, they are self-righteous. They have no goals and are aggressive. When things go as planned, they may become arrogant and lazy. Taeyangin also tend to be idealists (理想家) who dream of 'paradise' (武陵桃源). When their reality is different from their ideal, they are often discouraged, become lazy and resort to drinking alcohol for comfort. Therefore, Taeyangin should always cultivate their geungan (勤幹: diligent and incorrupt) and avoid alcohol and disinclination. This does mean avoiding all alcohol (禁酒), but when alcohol is consumed, it is important for Taeyangin to drink with good friends who understand them so that they can reach a state of moderation (中庸).

② Soyangin

Soyangin are active and passionate but hasty and careless. Soyangin have warm hearts. They are not calculative but tend to help others in need. They have a strong sense of justice. They are active in their social lives and love to stand out in the presence of others. However, Soyangin have a tendency to neglect themselves and their families. They have a tendency to exaggerate themselves in the presence of others. They like to impress others by clothing themselves in expensive materials (嬌奢), and they have strong sexual desires (好色), which may result in them neglecting their family. Sexual desires (好色) are not confined to enjoying sexual intercourse, but more broadly refer to an extravagant lifestyle that is not appropriate for one's income. To avoid these problems, Soyangin should simplify and minimize their lives (簡約) to stop extravagant overspending (驕奢).

③Taeeumin

Taeeumin are honest and reserved. They are trustworthy and are hardworking with strong perseverance. They are generally very conservative and are skeptical about change. They are always in doubt and conceal their true feelings. In other people's eyes, they may appear cunning and arrogant. Taeeumin are avaricious. They prioritize family matters over matters outside the home. They are not active and are somewhat lazy. If they have a strong lust for possessions, it can develop into greed (貪慾), and they may obsess over money or material possessions. Such greed (貪慾) can be overcome through listening and seeing (聞見). Listening and seeing refers to reading books, listening to lectures, traveling, and focusing on things other than themselves.

④ Soeumin

Soeumin are kind, calm and sociable, meticulous and good planners. They attend to small details and understand other people's feelings. Introverted in nature, Soeumin are generally very shy and do not express themselves. They are somewhat passive, so they do not actively pursue matters. Soeumin do not tolerate unsolicited advice and can become easily jealous. When they are emotionally hurt, they keep it inside for a long time. They are perceived as timid by others. They are quite calculative and like to group together people who they favor (Dangyeo; 黨與). Soeumin pursue authority and power (權勢). They do not extend their love to everyone, but are very selective of their peers. They enjoy power, whether it is a little or a lot, and they do not like to be controlled by others. They like to be in charge. Soeumin who are focused on authority and power (權勢) dislike being told what to do and are always jealous of others who have prominent abilities. They should keep this jealousy under control.

In common practice, when discussing the different constitutions, beneficial/harmful foods and herbal medications are usually referenced without acknowledging other factors. True Sasang medicine extends beyond the foods/medicines that are good for a specific type of person.

Sasang constitutional medicine perceives humans as physically and spiritually imperfect. Because humans are born imperfect, problems arise, and life can be perceived as a long process of solving these problems and pondering how to overcome these issues. Humans need to maintain a healthy lifestyle, both physically and spiritually. They need to be a part of society and have peers. This is related to how one adapts nature to reality. The phrase 'humans are born unwhole' suggests that, in physical terms, humans have constitutional differences in the size of the viscera. In mental terms, there are individual differences in states of real purpose (恒心: thoughts that are kept in the mind) and the inclination of the mind (心慾: greed that surfaces when the mind and nature are not properly controlled).

Dr. Je-Ma Lee wrote, 'The size (function) of the viscera in saints are no different from those of common people, but the size of their greed cause discrepancies between common people and saints.' In other words, humans have four natures (性), which are good: humanity, justice, propriety, and wisdom (仁義禮智). They also have four types of greed: rudeness, shallowness, greed, and indolence (鄙薄貪懶). Those who have more natures (性) are saints, and those who have more greeds (慾) are common people. Therefore, depending on how well the inclination of mind (心慾) is controlled and how well thoughts and actions (知行) are cultivated, one can become a saint or a commoner. When people can overcome their weaknesses and construct stronger thoughts and actions (知行) they can become saints.

Je-Ma Lee's definition of self-regulation does not end with cultivating one's mind, as is recommended by Daoism and Buddhism. It is based on Confucianist ideas that suggest, 'Cultivate oneself. Bring order to the family. Govern the country. Bring peace to all.' (修身齊家治國平天下). He emphasized that one should take care of oneself and family, as well as the entire society.

Je-Ma Lee emphasized the importance of abstinence from alcohol (酒), sex (色), wealth (財) and power (權) but also established guidelines for self-control.

Finally, Je-Ma Lee wrote, 'the worst thing to do in the world is to envy kind people and to be jealous of others' talents. The best thing to do in the world is to honor kind people and to enjoy doing kind things.' Envying kind people and being jealous of others' talents is a severe illness, while honoring kind people and enjoying doing kind things is a very effective medicine, which emphasizes the importance of mind control.

Therefore, Sasang medicine is not only a form of medicine, but a form of anthropology in that it focuses on 'what humans are and what they should pursue.'

By controlling and nurturing based on these principles, the mind and body can both become healthy. It is important to know one's Sasang constitution and the advantages and setbacks for each type. Changing lifestyles to better suit the constitutional type will lead to a healthy and happy life.

Appendix: Sasang Constitution Questionnaire

This questionnaire was developed to help determine your Sasang consitutional type.

Select the answer choices you consider best describes you. After you are done, find the diagnosis table at the back of the packet and check the appropriate boxes to find out what your Sasang type is.

▣ Example

Check(✓) the items of the survey and circle (○) the respective item on the table

Questionnaire 1. Which of the following statements describe your body frame?
① I have a large frame. ② Average. ③ I have a small frame.

↓

Table

Number		Constitution			
1	①			Taeeumin	
	②				
	③	Taeyangin○			Soeumin○

☞ If none describe you, omit the question. If one item describes you circle one item. If multiple items describe you, circle all that applies

■ Check the number for the item that applies to you.

1. Which of the following statements describes your body frame?
① I have a large frame. ② Average. ③ I have a small frame.

2. Which of the following statements describes your body form?
① I am large. ② I am about average. ③ I am small.

3. Which of the following statements describes your body proportion?
① The upper body is larger than the lower body.
② The lower body is larger than the upper body.
③ The upper body and the lower body are about the same proportion.

4. Which of the following statements describes your body?
① I have a well-developed neck area and a rather weak low back area.

② I have a well-developed chest area and rather weak buttocks area.
③ I have a well-developed low back area and a rather weak neck area.
④ I have well-developed buttocks and a rather weak chest area.

5. Which of the following statements describes your bone structure and overall features?
① Large bone structure and overweight
② Small bone structure and skinny
③ Average bone structure with a well-developed physique

6. Which of the following statements describe your chest?
① Broad and well-developed. (obesity type)
② Very thin and hunched. (slender)
③ Broad and strong. (muscular type)
④ Broad and sturdy.

7. What food temperature do you prefer?
① Warm food ② Cold food

8. Which of the following statements describe you?
① I have cold hands and feet. ② I have warm hands and feet.

9. Which of the following statements describe your walking habits?
① I walk slowly with dignity. ② I walk naturally and gently.
③ I walk briskly and swing my body back and forth.
④ I walk stiffly.

10. Which of the following statements describes you?
① I usually sweat a lot. I feel refreshed after I sweat.
② I do not usually sweat a lot. I feel tired after sweating.
③ I am not very tired after I sweat.

11. Which of the following statements describes you?
① outspoken and decisive ② active and courageous
③ dignified and formal ④ docile and sincere

12. Which of the following statements describes you? (in work or everyday activities)
① I do not withdraw no matter what. I move forward.
② I start projects but cannot finish them.
③ I prefer to work alone as opposed to moving around.
④ I tend to stay in one place and do not like to go out.

■ **Read the following statements carefully, and check only the ones that you feel describe your usual thoughts or actions.**

13. I take care of all matters very energetically.

14. I am very active and have strong will power.

15. I am not very calculating before I take action.

16. I can stay in a fixed place for a long time.

17. I am meticulous and careful.

18. I restrict my social activities to those with close friends.

19. I befriend others quite easily, without thinking much about it.

20. I am more focused on personal matters than social matters.

21. I think that appearance is more important than internal values.

22. I cannot befriend others easily because I am reserved in my thoughts.

23. I am neat and careful.

24. I am outspoken.

25. I am very sweet. I can comfort others well.

26. I am happy to participate in social events.

27. When I look at someone, I can tell whether or not he/she is diligent.

28. I am always in a hurry.

29. I am not comfortable speaking to strangers.

30. I am timid and always anxious.

31. I am usually quite sensitive.

32. I am patient.

33. I am quite careless.

34. I am swift and courageous.

35. I am more masculine than feminine.

36. I am bothered by small things.

37. I find it difficult to speak or present in front of others.

38. I am usually cheerful but have mood swings.

39. I pretend to be okay even when I am hurt.

40. When someone looks down on me, I cannot contain my anger.

41. I do not speak until I am sure that I am right.

42. I often pretend to know or boast about my knowledge.

43. I tend to neglect myself but am very polite to others.

44. I cannot take action in the presence of others.

45. I am not generous when returning favors to others.

46. I am often timid and anxious.

47. I am more feminine than masculine.

48. I have a desire to achieve more, even after I have achieved a considerable goal.

49. Sometimes I have vomited food or have not been able to swallow food for no specific reason.

50. When I am not well, sweating makes me feel better.

51. When I am not well, I have bad digestion.

52. I am usually very low in energy. I sigh a lot.

53. I have experienced several episodes of not being able to move my body, especially my legs, because I felt so low in energy.

54. I frequently feel uneasy in the chest and stomach after eating.

Table

Number		Constitution			
1	①			Taeeumin	
	②				
	③	Taeyangin			Soeumin
2	①			Taeeumin	
	②	Taeyangin	Soyangin		
	③				Soeumin
3	①			Taeeumin	
	②				Soeumin
	③		Soyangin		
4	①				
	②		Soyangin		
	③				
	④				Soeumin

Number		Constitution			
5	①			Taeeumin	
	②				Soeumin
	③		Soyangin		
6	①			Taeeumin	
	②				Soeumin
	③		Soyangin		
	④				
7	①				Soeumin
	②				
8	①				Soeumin
	②			Taeeumin	
9	①			Taeeumin	
	②				Soeumin
	③		Soyangin		
	④				
10	①			Taeeumin	
	②				Soeumin
	③				
11	①	Taeyangin			
	②			Taeeumin	
	③		Soyangin		
	④				Soeumin
12	①	Taeyangin			
	②		Soyangin		
	③				Soeumin
	④				

Number	Constitution			
13		Soyangin		
14		Soyangin	Taeeumin	
15		Soyangin		
16			Taeeumin	Soeumin
17				Soeumin
18				Soeumin
19		Soyangin		
20				Soeumin

Number	Constitution			
21	Taeyangin			
22			Taeeumin	
23				Soeumin
24	Taeyangin	Soyangin		
25				Soeumin
26			Taeeumin	
27			Taeeumin	
28		Soyangin		
29				Soeumin
30				Soeumin
31				Soeumin
32			Taeeumin	Soeumin
33		Soyangin		
34	Taeyangin			
35		Soyangin	Taeeumin	
36				Soeumin
37				Soeumin
38		Soyangin		
39				Soeumin
40	Taeyangin			
41				Soeumin
42		Soyangin		
43		Soyangin		
44				Soeumin
45	Taeyangin			
46				Soeumin
47				Soeumin
48	Taeyangin			
49	Taeyangin			
50			Taeeumin	
51				Soeumin
52				Soeumin
53				Soeumin
54				Soeumin
results	total ( )questions	total ( )questions	total ( )questions	total ( )questions
	(/11= %)	(/19= %)	(/17= %)	(/33= %)

How to evaluate the results

Of the 54 questions on this survey, 11 reflect Taeyangin traits, 19 for Soyangin, 17 for Taeeumin, and 33 for Soeumin traits. None of the questions refer to any two types. Some questions do not indicate a specific type.

One checked response counts as 1 point. Add up the scores for each constitution type and divide the number of answers you responded 'yes' to by the number of questions to obtain a percent (%). This value will be used to determine your Sasang type. The type that has the highest percentage value is your Sasang type, but only when the percentage score for that type is at least 10% higher than those for the other types. If not, the result is not significant.

The one exception is Taeyangin. To be a Taeyangin, the percentage score should be above 60%, and the difference between scores, as opposed to other types, should be at least 20%.

This test alone is not sufficient for identifying your Sasang type. If the results are ambiguous or if you want more information, visit a doctor of Korean medicine for consultation.

Example1) If you chose 1 Taeyangin item, 4 Soyangin items, 4 Taeeumin items, and 17 Soeumin items, Your percentage scores are 5% for Taeyangin (1/11), 20% for Soyangin (4/19), 25% for Taeeumin (4/17), and 50% for Soeumin (17/33). This means that you are a Soeumin-constitutional person. Your score for Soeumin is at least 25% higher than scores for other Sasang types. So you can be considered a Soeumin.

Sasang types	Constitution			
	Taeyangin	Soyangin	Taeeumin	Soeumin
results	total (1) questions	total (4) questions	total (4) questions	total (17) questions
	1/11=5%	4/19=20%	4/17=25%	17/33=50%

Example2) If your results indicate 70% Taeyangin, 40% Soyangin, 10% Taeeumin, and 30% Soeumin, you are a Taeyangin. However, if you are 60% Taeyangin, 50% Soyangin, 10% Taeeumin, and 20% Soeumin 20%, you cannot be considered a Taeyangin because the difference is not significant. (should be at least 20% difference)

Symptomatological Collection of Prescriptions in Korea's Sasang Medicine

1. Symptomatological Collection of Prescriptions in Korea's Sasang Medicine 東醫四象用藥彙分

1) Wind

Symptom	Taeeum type	Soeum type	Soyang type
Wind stroke	TE9 調胃續命湯 Stomach-Regulating Life-Prolonging Decoction	SE9 川芎桂枝湯 Cnidii Rhizoma and Cinnamomi Ramulus Decoction SE13 八物君子湯 Eight-Element Noble Decoction	SY8 獨活地黃湯 Angelicae Pubescentis Radix and Rehmanniae Radix Preparata Decoction SY9 荊防地黃湯 Schizonepetae, Saposhnikoviae, and Rehmanniae Radix Preparata Decoction
Bowels stroke	TE9 調胃續命湯 Stomach-Regulating Life-Prolonging Decoction	SE16 獨蔘八物湯 Ginseng-Emphasized Eight-Element Decoction SE2 人蔘桂枝附子湯 Ginseng, Cinnamomi Ramulus, and Aconiti Decoction	SY8 獨活地黃湯 Angelicae Pubescentis Radix and Rehmanniae Radix Preparata Decoction SY9 荊防地黃湯 Schizonepetae, Saposhnikoviae, and Rehmanniae Radix Preparata Decoction
Anuria and constipation due to bowels stroke	TE19 淸肺瀉肝湯 Lung-Clearing Liver-Purging Decoction TE59 二門五味湯 Liriope, Asparagus, and Schisandrae Decoction	SE31 巴豆丹 Crotonis Semen Pellet SE16 獨蔘八物湯 Ginseng-Emphasized Eight-Element Decoction SE36 官桂附子理中湯 Cinnamomi Cortex and Aconiti Lateralis Preparata Radix Middle-Regulating Decoction	SY28 輕粉甘隧龍虎丹 Calomelas and Euphorbiae Kansui Radix Dragon-Tiger Pellet SY18 地黃白虎湯 Rehmanniae Radix Crudus White Tiger Decoction
Bowels and viscera stroke	TE19 淸肺瀉肝湯 Lung-Clearing Liver-Purging Decoction TE50 二聖救苦丸	SE31 巴豆丹 Crotonis Semen Pellet SE36 官桂附子理中湯 Cinnamomi Cortex and	SY28 輕粉甘隧龍虎丹 Calomelas and Euphorbiae Kansui Radix Dragon-Tiger Pellet

Symptom	Taeeum type	Soeum type	Soyang type
	Two Holy Suffering-Saving Pill	Aconiti Lateralis Preparata Radix Middle-Regulating Decoction	SY14 降火地黃湯 Fire-Lowering Rehmanniae Radix Preparata Decoction
Emergency	TE45 牛黃淸心元 Bovis Calculus Heart-Clearing Pill TE55 滾痰湯 Phlegm-Sluicing Decoction TE39 瓜蒂散 Melonis Calyx Powder	SE55 蘇合香元 Styrax Liquides Pill SE16 獨蔘八物湯 Ginseng-Emphasized Eight-Element Decoction SE50 四逆湯 Four Counterflow Decoction	SY9 荊防地黃湯 Schizonepetae, Saposhnikoviae, and Rehmanniae Radix Preparata Decoction SY48 靈砂散 Vermilionum Powder SY8 獨活地黃湯 Angelicae Pubescentis Radix and Rehmanniae Radix Preparata Decoction
Deviated eye and mouth	TE1 太陰調胃湯 Taeeum Stomach-Regulating Decoction	SE21 祛風散 Wind-Dispelling Powder SE82 牽正散 Deviation-Correcting Powder	SY8 獨活地黃湯 Angelicae Pubescentis Radix and Rehmanniae Radix Preparata Decoction SY9 荊防地黃湯 Schizonepetae, Saposhnikoviae, and Rehmanniae Radix Preparata Decoction
Tetanus	TE62 三黃散 Three Yellows Powder	SE88 如神湯 Marvelous Decoction	SY30 乳香沒藥輕粉丸 Olibanum, Myrrha, and Calomelas Pill
Nose and forehead pain	TE53 如神炷 Marvelous Incense Stick	SE9 川芎桂枝湯 Cnidii Rhizoma and Cinnamomi Ramulus Decoction	SY1 荊防敗毒散 Schizonepetae Spica and Saposhnikoviae Radix Toxin-Repelling Powder
Hemiplegia	TE1 太陰調胃湯 Taeeum Stomach-Regulating Decoction TE12 調胃升淸湯 Stomach-Regulating Upraising-Clearing Decoction	SE15 十全大補湯 Ten Wholesome Greatly Tonifying Decoction SE13 八物君子湯 Eight-Element Noble Decoction SE83 唐橘湯 Rubi Flos and Citri Fructus Preparata Decoction	SY8 獨活地黃湯 Angelicae Pubescentis Radix and Rehmanniae Radix Preparata Decoction SY9 荊防地黃湯 Schizonepetae, Saposhnikoviae, and Rehmanniae Radix Preparata Decoction
Phlegm exuberance	TE1 太陰調胃湯 Taeeum	SE54 木香順氣散 Aucklandiae Radix	SY40 李氏凉膈散 Lee's Diaphragm-Cooling

Symptom	Taeeum type	Soeum type	Soyang type
	Stomach-Regulating Decoction TE26 萊菔子承氣湯 Raphani Semen Qi-Coordinating Decoction	Qi-Arranging Powder SE21 祛風散 Wind-Dispelling Powder	Powder SY20 凉膈散火湯 Diaphragm-Cooling Fire-Dissipating Decoction
Heat syndrome	TE35 藁本浮萍湯 Angelicae Tenuissimae Radix and Spirodelae Herba Decoction	SE13 八物君子湯 Eight-Element Noble Decoction	SY20 凉膈散火湯 Diaphragm-Cooling Fire-Dissipating Decoction
Deficiency syndrome	TE1 太陰調胃湯 Taeeum Stomach-Regulating Decoction TE12 調胃升淸湯 Stomach-Regulating Upraising-Clearing Decoction	SE13 八物君子湯 Eight-Element Noble Decoction	SY9 荊防地黃湯 Schizonepetae, Saposhnikoviae, and Rehmanniae Radix Preparata Decoction
Qi regulating	TE15 淸心蓮子湯 Heart-Clearing Nelumbinis Semen Decoction	SE55 蘇合香元 Styrax Liquides Pill SE23 赤白何烏寬中湯 Polygoni Multiflori Radix and Cynanchi Wilfordii Radix Middle-Soothing Decoction	SY41 六味地黃湯 Six-Element Rehmanniae Radix Preparata Decoction
In general	TE12 調胃升淸湯 Stomach-Regulating Upraising-Clearing Decoction	SE15 十全大補湯 Ten Wholesome Greatly Tonifying Decoction	SY9 荊防地黃湯 Schizonepetae, Saposhnikoviae, and Rehmanniae Radix Preparata Decoction
Moving impediment	TE9 調胃續命湯 Stomach-Regulating Life-Prolonging Decoction	SE10 芎歸香蘇散 Cnidii, Angelicae Gigantis, Cyperi, and Perillae Powder	SY1 荊防敗毒散 Schizonepetae Spica and Saposhnikoviae Radix Toxin-Repelling Powder
Akinesia	TE9 調胃續命湯 Stomach-Regulating Life-Prolonging Decoction TE35 藁本浮萍湯 Angelicae Tenuissimae Radix and Spirodelae Herba Decoction	SE21 祛風散 Wind-Dispelling Powder SE83 唐橘湯 Rubi Flos and Citri Fructus Preparata Decoction	SY28 輕粉甘隧龍虎丹 Calomelas and Euphorbiae Kansui Radix Dragon-Tiger Pellet
Loss of voice	TE45 牛黃淸心元 Bovis Calculus Heart-Clearing Pill	SE84 壽脾解語湯 Spleen-Longevity Speech-Releasing	SY54 歸腎解語散 Kidney-Restoring Speech-Releasing

Symptom	Taeeum type	Soeum type	Soyang type
	TE56 祛風解語散 Wind-Dispelling Speech-Releasing Powder	Decoction	Decoction
Joint-runnung wind	TE19 清肺瀉肝湯 加蒼芪 Lung-Clearing Liver-Purging Decoction added Atractylodis Rhizoma and Astragali Radix	SE21 祛風散 Wind-Dispelling Powder	SY20 凉膈散火湯 Diaphragm-Cooling Fire-Dissipating Decoction SY31 輕粉乳香沒藥丸 Calomelas, Olibanum, and Myrrha Pill
Skin rashes	TE11 葛根解肌湯 Puerariae Radix Flesh-Resolving Decoction TE19 清肺瀉肝湯 Lung-Clearing Liver-Purging Decoction	SE21 祛風散 Wind-Dispelling Powder SE6 補中益氣湯 Middle-Tonifying Qi-Replenishing Decoction SE15 十全大補湯 Ten Wholesome Greatly Tonifying Decoction	SY20 凉膈散火湯 Diaphragm-Cooling Fire-Dissipating Decoction SY46 消毒飮 Toxin-Dissolving Decoction
Sudden aphasia	TE40 熊膽散 Fel Ursi Powder TE9 調胃續命湯 Stomach-Regulating Life-Prolonging Decoction	SE15 十全大補湯 Ten Wholesome Greatly Tonifying Decoction SE16 獨蔘八物湯 Ginseng-Emphasized Eight-Element Decoction	SY20 凉膈散火湯 Diaphragm-Cooling Fire-Dissipating Decoction SY40 李氏凉膈散 Lee's Diaphragm-Cooling Powder

2) Cold

Symptom	Taeeum type	Soeum type	Soyang type
Greater yang syndrome	TE28 麻黃發表湯 Ephedrae Herba Exterior-Effusing Decoction TE9 調胃續命湯 Stomach-Regulating Life-Prolonging Decoction	腎熱: SE9 川芎桂枝湯 Kidney heat: Cnidii Rhizoma and Cinnamomi Ramulus Decoction SE13 八物君子湯 Eight-Element Noble Decoction Aversion to cold: SE91 藿香正氣散 Agastachis Herba Qi-Correcting Powder, SE22 香砂養胃湯 Cyperi Rhizoma and Amomi Fructus Stomach-	SY1 荊防敗毒散 Schizonepetae Spica and Saposhnikoviae Radix Toxin-Repelling Powder Severe : SY4 荊防瀉白散 Schizonepetae Spica and Saposhnikoviae Radix White-Draining Powder

Symptom	Taeeum type	Soeum type	Soyang type
		Nourishing Decoction, SE10 芎歸香蘇散 Cnidii, Angelicae Gigantis, Cyperi, and Perillae Powder Discharging deficiency: SE91 藿香正氣散 Agastachis Herba Qi-Correcting Powder	
Continuous fever due to epidemic cold	TE21 寒多熱少湯 Cold-Dominant Heat-Recessive Decoction TE8 升芩調胃湯 Cimicifugae Rhizoma and Scutellariae Radix Stomach-Regulating Decoction	Reverting yin: SE35 人蔘吳茱萸湯 Ginseng Radix and Evodiae Fructus Decoction SE16 獨蔘八物湯 Ginseng-Emphasized Eight-Element Decoction	Interior syndrome like malaria : SY6 猪苓車前子湯 Polyporus and Plantaginis Semen Decoction Constipation : SY4 荊防瀉白散
	TE40 熊膽散 Fel Ursi powder 菖蒲透邪湯 Acori Graminei Rhizoma Pathogen-Outthrusting Decoction Heat : TE6 承氣調胃湯 Qi-Coordinating Stomach- Regulating Decoction TE23 潤肺淸肝湯 Lung-Moistening Liver-Clearing Decoction		Schizonepetae Spica and Saposhnikoviae Radix White-Draining Powder
Yang brightness syndrome	TE11 葛根解肌湯 Puerariae Radix Flesh-Resolving Decoction	SE13 八物君子湯 Eight-Element Noble Decoction SE5 升陽益氣湯 Yang-Upraising Qi-Replenishing Decoction	SY1 荊防敗毒散 Schizonepetae Spica and Saposhnikoviae Radix Toxin-Repelling Powder Worse : SY44 李氏導赤散 Lee's Red-Conducting Powder Steaming bone and Sweating : SY2 荊防導赤散 Schizonepetae Spica and Saposhnikoviae Radix Red-Conducting Powder SY6 猪苓車前子湯 Polyporus and Plantaginis Semen

Symptom	Taeeum type	Soeum type	Soyang type
			Decoction SY18 地黃白虎湯 Rehmanniae Radix Crudus White Tiger Decoction
Lesser yang syndrome	TE18 熱多寒少湯 Heat-Dominant Cold-Recessive Decoction	SE91 藿香正氣散 Agastachis Herba Qi-Correcting Powder	SY1 荊防敗毒散 Schizonepetae Spica and Saposhnikoviae Radix Toxin-Repelling Powder
		SE22 香砂養胃湯 Cyperi Rhizoma and Amomi Fructus Stomach-Nourishing Decoction	SY4 荊防瀉白散 Schizonepetae Spica and Saposhnikoviae Radix White-Draining Powder Constipation: SY18 地黃白虎湯 Rehmanniae Radix Crudus White Tiger Decoction
Greater yin syndrome	Cold pattern : TE1 太陰調胃湯 Taeeum Stomach-Regulating Decoction Heat pattern : TE11 葛根解肌湯 Puerariae Radix Flesh-Resolving Decoction	SE43 白何烏理中湯 Cynanchi Wilfordii Radix Middle-Regulating Decoction SE42 白何烏附子理中湯 Cynanchi Wilfordii Radix and Aconiti Lateralis Radix Preparata Middle-Regulating Decoction Yin toxin syndrome: SE33 人蔘陳皮湯 Ginseng Radix and Citri Unshius Pericarpium SE34 人蔘桂皮湯 Ginseng Radix and Cinnamomi Cortex Decoction	Yin damage due to fever : SY9 荊防地黃湯 Schizonepetae, Saposhnikoviae, and Rehmanniae Radix Preparata Decoction SY6 猪苓車前子湯 Polyporus and Plantaginis Semen Decoction
Lesser yin syndrome	TE18 熱多寒少湯 Heat-Dominant Cold-Recessive Decoction	SE36 官桂附子理中湯 Cinnamomi Cortex and Aconiti Lateralis Preparata Radix Middle-Regulating Decoction SE40 吳茱萸附子理中湯 Evodiae Fructus and Aconiti Lateralis Radix Preparata Middle-Regulating Decoction	SY18 地黃白虎湯 Rehmanniae Radix Crudus White Tiger Decoction Yin damage due to fever : SY7 滑石苦蔘湯 Talcum and Sophorae Radix Decoction

Symptom	Taeeum type	Soeum type	Soyang type
Half-exterior half-interior syndrome	TE6 承氣調胃湯 Qi-Coordinating Stomach-Regulating Decoction	SE9 川芎桂枝湯 Cnidii Rhizoma and Cinnamomi Ramulus Decoction SE91 藿香正氣散 Agastachis Herba Qi-Correcting Powder	SY55 新小柴胡湯 New Bupleuri Radix Minor Decoction SY4 荊防瀉白散 Schizonepetae Spica and Saposhnikoviae Radix White-Draining Powder
Manic onset	TE25 葛根大承氣湯 Puerariae Radix Major Qi-Coordinating Decoction TE26 萊菔子承氣湯 Raphani Semen Qi-Coordinating Decoction	SE16 獨蔘八物湯 Ginseng-Emphasized Eight-Element Decoction	SY56 新大柴胡湯 New Bupleuri Radix Major Decoction Exterior syndrome of constipation after diarrhea : SY32 白虎湯 White Tiger Decoction SY58 降陰白虎湯 Yin-Lowering White Tiger Decoction
Delirious speech	TE25 葛根大承氣湯 Puerariae Radix Major Qi-Coordinating Decoction	Choose and use the appropriate one among prescriptions for Soeum type in the Cold part.	Yang brightness pattern : SY18 地黃白虎湯 Rehmanniae Radix Crudus White Tiger Decoction Lesser yang pattern : SY56 新大柴胡湯 New Bupleuri Radix Major Decoction Yin collapse pattern : Choose and use the one among four yin- collapse related prescriptions.
Stuffiness	TE26 萊菔子承氣湯 Raphani Semen Qi-Coordinating Decoction	SE31 巴豆丹 Crotonis Semen Pellet SE91 藿香正氣散 Agastachis Herba Qi-Correcting Powder	Abdominal pain : SY7 滑石苦蔘湯 Talcum and Sophorae Radix Decoction SY-e22 贊化丹 Transformation-Helping Pellet
			SY9 荊防地黃湯 Schizonepetae, Saposhnikoviae, and Rehmanniae Radix Preparata Decoction
Vomiting ascariasis	TE18 熱多寒少湯 Heat-Dominant	SE47 理中湯 Middle-Regulating	The treatment is similar to that of chest bind.

Symptom	Taeeum type	Soeum type	Soyang type
	Cold-Recessive Decoction	Decoction SE42 白何烏附子理中湯 Cynanchi Wilfordii Radix and Aconiti Lateralis Radix Preparata Middle-Regulating Decoction	Choose and use the one among four yin-collapse-related prescriptions.
Chest bind	TE66 李氏承氣湯 Lee's Qi-Coordinating Decoction	SE20 桂枝半夏生薑湯 Cinnamomi, Pinelliae, and Zingiberis Decoction SE23 赤白何烏寬中湯 Polygoni Multiflori Radix and Cynanchi Wilfordii Radix Middle-Soothing Decoction SE31 巴豆丹 Crotonis Semen Pellet	SY3 導赤降氣湯 Red-Conducting Qi-Lowering Decoction Delirium : SY18 地黃白虎湯 Rehmanniae Radix Crudus White Tiger Decoction SY52 大甘遂散 Euphorbiae Kansui Radix Major Powder SY53 小甘遂散 Euphorbiae Kansui Radix Minor Powder
Cold stroke	TE1 太陰調胃湯 Taeeum Stomach-Regulating Decoction	SE42 白何烏附子理中湯 Cynanchi Wilfordii Radix and Aconiti Lateralis Radix Preparata Middle-Regulating Decoction	SY7 滑石苦蔘湯 Talcum and Sophorae Radix Decoction
Pestilence	Not even one (disease) is not a six-meridian disease. It should be treated according to six meridian divisions.		

3) Summerheat

Symptom	Taeeum type	Soeum type	Soyang type
Summerheat stroke	TE49 生脈散 Pulse-Activating Powder	SE38 桂附藿陳理中湯 Cinnamomi, Aconiti, Agastachis, and Citri Unshius Middle-Regulating Decoction SE43 白何烏理中湯 Cynanchi Wilfordii Radix Middle-Regulating Decoction	SY26 朱砂益元散 Cinnabaris Prime-Replenishing Powder

Symptom	Taeeum type	Soeum type	Soyang type
Summerheat stagnation	TE15 淸心蓮子湯 Heart-Clearing Nelumbinis Semen Decoction TE26 萊菔子承氣湯 Raphani Semen Qi-Coordinating Decoction	SE38 桂附藿陳理中湯 Cinnamomi, Aconiti, Agastachis, and Citri Unshius Middle-Regulating Decoction	SY27 甘遂天一丸 Euphorbiae Kansui Radix Heaven-One Pill
Vexing thirst	TE49 生脈散 Pulse-Activating Powder TE11 葛根解肌湯 Puerariae Radix Flesh-Resolving Decoction	SE43 白何烏理中湯 Cynanchi Wilfordii Radix Middle-Regulating Decoction SY61 三味蔘萸湯 Three-Flavor Ginseng Radix and Evodiae Fructus Decoction	SY26 朱砂益元散 Cinnabaris Prime-Replenishing Powder
Vomiting and diarrhea	TE18 熱多寒少湯 Heat-Dominant Cold-Recessive Decoction Poisoning : TE41 麝香散 Moschus Decoction	SE24 十二味寬中湯 Twelve-Flavor Middle-Soothing Decoction SY61 三味蔘萸湯 Three-Flavor Ginseng Radix and Evodiae Fructus Decoction	SY6 猪苓車前子湯 Polyporus and Plantaginis Semen Decoction

4) Dampness

	Taeeum type	Soeum type	Soyang type
In general	Cold: TE10 腎氣調胃湯 Kidney Qi Stomach-Regulating Decoction Heat: TE6 承氣調胃湯 : Qi-Coordinating Stomach-Regulating Decoction	SE45 寬中湯 Middle-Soothing Decoction	SY6 猪苓車前子湯 Polyporus and Plantaginis Semen Decoction

5) Dryness

	Taeeum type	Soeum type	Soyang type
In general	TE19 淸肺瀉肝湯 Lung-Clearing Liver-Purging Decoction	SE13 八物君子湯 Eight-Element Noble Decoction	SY20 凉膈散火湯 Diaphragm-Cooling Fire-Dissipating Decoction

6) Fire

Symptom	Taeeum type	Soeum type	Soyang type
Heat	TE19 清肺瀉肝湯 Lung-Clearing Liver-Purging Decoction	SE13 八物君子湯 Eight-Element Noble Decoction	SY20 凉膈散火湯 Diaphragm-Cooling Fire-Dissipating Decoction
Steaming bone	TE1 太陰調胃湯 Taeeum Stomach-Regulating Decoction TE15 淸心蓮子湯 Heart-Clearing Nelumbinis Semen Decoction	SE6 補中益氣湯 Middle-Tonifying Qi-Replenishing Decoction	SY17 十二味地黃湯 Twelve-Flavor Rehmanniae Radix Preparata Decoction SY8 獨活地黃湯 Angelicae Pubescentis Radix and Rehmanniae Radix Preparata Decoction

7) Internal damage

	Taeeum type	Soeum type	Soyang type
Food damage	TE1 太陰調胃湯 Taeeum Stomach-Regulating Decoction	SE22 香砂養胃湯 Cyperi Rhizoma and Amomi Fructus Stomach- Nourishing Decoction	SY20 凉膈散火湯 Diaphragm-Cooling Fire-Dissipating Decoction
Phlegm stagnation	TE1 太陰調胃湯 Taeeum Stomach-Regulating Decoction	SE22 香砂養胃湯 Cyperi Rhizoma and Amomi Fructus Stomach- Nourishing Decoction	SY20 凉膈散火湯 Diaphragm-Cooling Fire-Dissipating Decoction
Cold stagnation	TE1 太陰調胃湯 Taeeum Stomach-Regulating Decoction	SE43 白何烏理中湯 Cynanchi Wilfordii Radix Middle-Regulating Decoction SE42 白何烏附子理中湯 Cynanchi Wilfordii Radix and Aconiti Lateralis Radix Preparata Middle-Regulating Decoction	SY20 凉膈散火湯 Diaphragm-Cooling Fire-Dissipating Decoction SY41 六味地黃湯 Six-Element Rehmanniae Radix Preparata Decoction
Retained stagnation	TE1 太陰調胃湯 Taeeum Stomach-Regulating Decoction	SE68 如意丹 Pliant Pellet	SY20 凉膈散火湯 Diaphragm-Cooling Fire-Dissipating Decoction

Symptom	Taeeum type	Soeum type	Soyang type
			SY41 六味地黃湯 Six-Element Rehmanniae Radix Preparata Decoction SY-e22 贊化丹 Transformation-Helping Pellet
Persistent fullness	TE15 淸心蓮子湯 Heart-Clearing Nelumbinis Semen Decoction TE12 調胃升淸湯 Stomach-Regulating Upraising-Clearing Decoction	SE69 香砂六君子湯 Cyperi Rhizoma and Amomi Fructus Six Noble Decoction SE6 補中益氣湯 Middle-Tonifying Qi-Replenishing Decoction	SY41 六味地黃湯 Six-Element Rehmanniae Radix Preparata Decoction SY9 荊防地黃湯 Schizonepetae, Saposhnikoviae, and Rehmanniae Radix Preparata Decoction
Loss of appetite	TE15 淸心蓮子湯 Heart-Clearing Nelumbinis Semen Decoction TE12 調胃升淸湯 Stomach-Regulating Upraising-Clearing Decoction	SE69 香砂六君子湯 Cyperi Rhizoma and Amomi Fructus Six Noble Decoction SE6 補中益氣湯 Middle-Tonifying Qi-Replenishing Decoction	SY41 六味地黃湯 Six-Element Rehmanniae Radix Preparata Decoction SY9 荊防地黃湯 Schizonepetae, Saposhnikoviae, and Rehmanniae Radix Preparata Decoction
Alcoholic damage	TE6 承氣調胃湯 去 大黃 Qi-Coordinating Stomach-Regulating Decoction removed Rhei Rhizoma	SE13 八物君子湯 Eight-Element Noble Decoction	SY41 六味地黃湯 Six-Element Rehmanniae Radix Preparata Decoction
Acid regurgitation	TE11 葛根解肌湯 Puerariae Radix Flesh-Resolving Decoction	SE22 香砂養胃湯 Cyperi Rhizoma and Amomi Fructus Stomach-Nourishing Decoction SE28 薑朮寬中湯 Zingiberis Rhizoma and Atractylodis Rhizoma Alba Middle-Soothing Decoction	SY20 凉膈散火湯 Diaphragm-Cooling Fire-Dissipating Decoction
Gastric upset and belching	TE11 葛根解肌湯 Puerariae Radix Flesh-Resolving Decoction	SE22 香砂養胃湯 Cyperi Rhizoma and Amomi Fructus Stomach-Nourishing Decoction	SY20 凉膈散火湯 Diaphragm-Cooling Fire-Dissipating Decoction

	Taeeum type	Soeum type	Soyang type
		SE28 薑朮寬中湯 Zingiberis Rhizoma and Atractylodis Rhizoma Alba Middle-Soothing Decoction	

8) Consumptive Disease

Symptom	Taeeum type	Soeum type	Soyang type
In general	TE1 太陰調胃湯 Taeeum Stomach-Regulating Decoction TE12 調胃升淸湯 Stomach-Regulating Upraising-Clearing Decoction TE31 拱辰黑元丹 Polaris-Aspiring Black Vitality Pellet TE32 鹿茸大補湯 Cervi Parvum Cornu Greatly Tonifying Decoction (Cervi Parvum Cornu 鹿茸 can be changed into Puerariae Surculus 葛茸.)	SE6 補中益氣湯 Middle-Tonifying Qi-Replenishing Decoction SE13 八物君子湯 Eight-Element Noble Decoction SE15 十全大補湯 Ten Wholesome Greatly Tonifying Decoction	SY41 六味地黃湯 Six-Element Rehmanniae Radix Preparata Decoction SY9 荊防地黃湯 Schizonepetae, Saposhnikoviae, and Rehmanniae Radix Preparata Decoction

9) Cholera and Gastroenteritis

Symptom	Taeeum type	Soeum type	Soyang type
In general	TE18 熱多寒少湯 Heat-Dominant Cold-Recessive Decoction Block and repulsion: TE11 葛根解肌湯 Puerariae Radix Flesh-Resolving Decoction	SE24 十二味寬中湯 Twelve-Flavor Middle-Soothing Decoction SY61 三味蔘萸湯 Three-Flavor Ginseng Radix and Evodiae Fructus Decoction SE38 桂附藿陳理中湯 Cinnamomi, Aconiti, Agastachis, and Citri Unshius	SY6 猪苓車前子湯 Polyporus and Plantaginis Semen Decoction Block and repulsion: SY27 甘遂天一丸 Euphorbiae Kansui Radix Heaven-One Pill

Symptom	Taeeum type	Soeum type	Soyang type
		Middle-Regulating Decoction Block and repulsion: SE31 巴豆丹 Crotonis Semen Pellet	
Vomitting and diarrhea	TE15 淸心蓮子湯 Heart-Clearing Nelumbinis Semen Decoction	SY61 三味蔘萸湯 Three-Flavor Ginseng Radix and Evodiae Fructus Decoction	SY41 六味地黃湯 Six-Element Rehmanniae Radix Preparata Decoction
Dry retching	TE15 淸心蓮子湯 Heart-Clearing Nelumbinis Semen Decoction	SE48 白何烏官桂理中湯 Cynanchi Wilfordii Radi and Cinnamomi Cortex Middle-Regulating Decoction SE20 桂枝半夏生薑湯 Cinnamomi, Pinelliae, and Zingiberis Decoction	SY41 六味地黃湯 Six-Element Rehmanniae Radix Preparata Decoction
Nausea	TE18 熱多寒少湯 (或加大黃) Heat-Dominant Cold-Recessive Decoction (or added Rhei Rhizoma)	SE48 白何烏官桂理中湯 Cynanchi Wilfordii Radi and Cinnamomi Cortex Middle-Regulating Decoction SE20 桂枝半夏生薑湯 Cinnamomi, Pinelliae, and Zingiberis Decoction SE34 人蔘桂皮湯 Ginseng Radix and Cinnamomi Cortex Decoction SE40 吳茱萸附子理中湯 Evodiae Fructus and Aconiti Lateralis Radix Preparata Middle-Regulating Decoction	SY20 凉膈散火湯 Diaphragm-Cooling Fire-Dissipating Decoction

10) Cough

Symptom	Taeeum type	Soeum type	Soyang type
In general	TE1 太陰調胃湯 Taeeum Stomach-Regulating Decoction	Cough due to overexertion : SE6 補中益氣湯 Middle-Tonifying	Cough due to overexertion : SY10 前胡地黃湯 Angelicae Decursivae Radix and

Symptom	Taeeum type	Soeum type	Soyang type
	TE32 鹿茸大補湯 Cervi Parvum Cornu Greatly Tonifying Decoction TE31 拱辰黑元丹 Polaris-Aspiring Black Vitality Pellet ◆ 葛茸大補湯 Puerariae Surculus Greatly Tonifying Decoction TE7 經驗調胃湯 Empirical Stomach-Regulating Decoction TE10 腎氣調胃湯 Kidney Qi Stomach-Regulating Decoction Dyspnea : TE16 麻黃定喘湯 Ephedrae Herba Panting-Stabilizing Decoction	Qi-Replenishing Decoction ◆ 李氏補中益氣湯 Lee's Middle-Tonifying Qi-Replenishing Decoction Cold-Cough : SE42 白何烏附子理中湯 Cynanchi Wilfordii Radix and Aconiti Lateralis Radix Preparata Middle-Regulating Decoction SE36 官桂附子理中湯 Cinnamomi Cortex and Aconiti Lateralis Preparata Radix Middle- Regulating Decoction Wind-cold : SE21 祛風散 Wind-Dispelling Powder Stagnation : SE24 十二味寬中湯 Twelve-Flavor Middle-Soothing Decoction Blood: SE6 補中益氣湯 Middle-Tonifying Qi-Replenishing Decoction SE15 十全大補湯 Ten Wholesome Greatly Tonifying Decoction	Rehmanniae Radix Preparata Decoction Cough due to Depression : SY4 荊防瀉白散 Schizonepetae Spica and Saposhnikoviae Radix White-Draining Powder Cough due to Fire: SY18 地黃白虎湯 Rehmanniae Radix Crudus White Tiger Decoction Symptoms due to liquor : SY9 荊防地黃湯 Schizonepetae, Saposhnikoviae, and Rehmanniae Radix Preparata Decoction Dyspnea: SY10 前胡地黃湯 Angelicae Decursivae Radix and Rehmanniae Radix Preparata Decoction added Trichosanthis Semen 瓜蔞仁. SY41 六味地黃湯 Six-Element Rehmanniae Radix Preparata Decoction

11) Aggregation-Accumulation

Symptom	Taeeum type	Soeum type	Soyang type
Six types of depression	Qi depression : TE15 淸心蓮子湯 Heart-Clearing Nelumbinis Semen Decoction	Qi depression: SE24 十二味寬中湯 Twelve-Flavor Middle-Soothing Decoction, SE71 保命飮 Life-Protecting Decoction	Qi depression: SY20 凉膈散火湯 Diaphragm-Cooling Fire-Dissipating Decoction

Symptom	Taeeum type	Soeum type	Soyang type
	Dampness depression : TE1 太陰調胃湯 Taeeum Stomach-Regulating Decoction Phlegm depression: TE18 熱多寒少湯 Heat-Dominant Cold-Recessive Decoction Heat depression: TE18 熱多寒少湯 Heat-Dominant Cold-Recessive Decoction TE19 淸肺瀉肝湯 Lung-Clearing Liver-Purging Decoction Draining depression: TE19 淸肺瀉肝湯 Lung-Clearing Liver-Purging Decoction Food depression: TE15 淸心蓮子湯 Heart-Clearing Nelumbinis Semen Decoction TE19 淸肺瀉肝湯 Lung-Clearing Liver-Purging Decoction	Dampness Depression: SE24 十二味寬中湯 Twelve-Flavor Middle-Soothing Decoction Phlegm Depression: SE24 十二味寬中湯 Twelve-Flavor Middle-Soothing Decoction SE21 祛風散 Wind-Dispelling Powder SE71 保命飮 Life-Protecting Decoction Heat depression: SE24 十二味寬中湯 Twelve-Flavor Middle-Soothing Decoction Blood depression: SE26 當歸白何烏寬中湯 Angelicae Gigantis Radix and Polygoni Multiflori Radix Alba Middle-Soothing Decoction Food depression: SE22 香砂養胃湯 Cyperi Rhizoma and Amomi Fructus Stomach-Nourishing Decoction	Dampness depression: SY9 荊防地黃湯 Schizonepetae, Saposhnikoviae, and Rehmanniae Radix Preparata Decoction Phlegm depression: SY20 凉膈散火湯 Diaphragm-Cooling Fire-Dissipating Decoction SY4 荊防瀉白散 Schizonepetae Spica and Saposhnikoviae Radix White-Draining Powder Heat depression: SY19 陽毒白虎湯 Yang Toxin White Tiger Decoction, SY21 忍冬藤地骨皮湯 Lonicerae Caulis and Lycii Radicis Cortex Decoction Blood depression: SY15 生熟地黃湯 Rehmanniae Radix Crudus et Preparata Decoction
Alcoholic accumulation	TE19 淸肺瀉肝湯 Lung-Clearing Liver-Purging Decoction	SE24 十二味寬中湯 Twelve-Flavor Middle-Soothing Decoction added Atractylodis Rhizoma 蒼朮 and removed Polygoni Multiflori Radix Alba 白何首烏	SY40 李氏凉膈散 Lee's Diaphragm-Cooling Powder
Fish and crab accumulations	TE1 太陰調胃湯 Taeeum Stomach-Regulating Decoction	SE56 香蘇散 Cyperi Rhizoma and Perillae Folium Powder	SY1 荊防敗毒散 加 連翹 牛蒡子 Schizonepetae Spica and Saposhnikoviae Radix Toxin-Repelling Powder

Symptom	Taeeum type	Soeum type	Soyang type
			added Forsythiae Fructus 連翹 and Arctii Fructus 牛蒡子
Fruit and vegetable accumulations	TE36 葛茸浮萍湯 Puerariae, Cervi Parvum Cornu, and Spirodelae Decoction	SE22 香砂養胃湯 Cyperi Rhizoma and Amomi Fructus Stomach-Nourishing Decoction	SY1 荊防敗毒散 加 神曲 麥芽 Schizonepetae Spica and Saposhnikoviae Radix Toxin-Repelling Powder added Massa Medicata Fermentata 神曲 and Hordei Fructus Germinatus 麥芽
Water accumulation	TE1 太陰調胃湯 Taeeum Stomach-Regulating Decoction TE19 淸肺瀉肝湯 Lung-Clearing Liver-Purging Decoction	SE24 十二味寬中湯 Twelve-Flavor Middle-Soothing Decoction SE45 寬中湯 Middle-Soothing Decoction	SY9 荊防地黃湯 Schizonepetae, Saposhnikoviae, and Rehmanniae Radix Preparata Decoction SY27 甘遂天一丸 Euphorbiae Kansui Radix Heaven-One Pill
Worm accumulation	TE17 麻黃定痛湯 Ephedrae Herba Pain-Stabilizing Decoction TE19 淸肺瀉肝湯 Lung-Clearing Liver-Purging Decoction	◆ 人蔘附子理中湯 Ginseng Radix and Aconiti Lateralis Radix Preparata Middle-Regulating Decoction	No lump : SY7 滑石苦蔘湯 Talcum and Sophorae Radix Decoction, SY45 李氏肥兒丸 Lee's Child-Plumping Pill
		SE42 白何烏附子理中湯 Cynanchi Wilfordii Radix and Aconiti Lateralis Radix Preparata Middle-Regulating Decoction	Lump : SY21 忍冬藤地骨皮湯 Lonicerae Caulis and Lycii Radicis Cortex Decoction
Aggregation-accumulation	TE18 熱多寒少湯 Heat-Dominant Cold-Recessive Decoction	◆ 人蔘附子理中湯 Ginseng Radix and Aconiti Lateralis Radix Preparata Middle-Regulating Decoction	SY21 忍冬藤地骨皮湯 Lonicerae Caulis and Lycii Radicis Cortex Decoction
In general	TE-e16 四時丹 Four seasons Pellet	SE31 巴豆丹 Crotonis Semen Pellet SE63 溫白元 White-Warming Pill SE68 如意丹 Pliant Pellet	SY-e22 贊化丹 Transformation-Helping Pellet

12) Puffy Swelling

Symptom	Taeeum type	Soeum type	Soyang type
Interior heat	TE34 葛根浮萍湯 Puerariae Radix and Spirodelae Herba Decoction	SE22 香砂養胃湯 Cyperi Rhizoma and Amomi Fructus Stomach-Nourishing Decoction SE39 芎歸葱蘇理中湯 Cnidii, Angelicae Gigantis, Allii Fistulosi, and Perillae Middle-Regulating Decoction	SY23 木通大安湯 Akebiae Caulis Greatly Relieving Decoction
Exterior cold	TE37 乾栗蠐螬湯 Castaneae Semen and Holotrichia Vermis Decoction	SE39 芎歸葱蘇理中湯 Cnidii, Angelicae Gigantis, Allii Fistulosi, and Perillae Middle-Regulating Decoction SE71 保命飮 Life-Protecting Decoction SE70 鎭陰膽 Yin-Suppressing Tartare SE24 十二味寬中湯 Twelve-Flavor Middle-Soothing Decoction	SY16 木通無憂湯 Akebiae Caulis Anxiety-Free Decoction

13) Distention and Fullness

Symptom	Taeeum type	Soeum type	Soyang type
Qi distention	TE1 太陰調胃湯 Taeeum Stomach-Regulating Decoction	SE24 十二味寬中湯 Twelve-Flavor Middle-Soothing Decoction	Deficiency: SY9 荊防地黃湯 Schizonepetae, Saposhnikoviae, and Rehmanniae Radix Preparata Decoction Fire: SY20 凉膈散火湯 Diaphragm-Cooling Fire-Dissipating Decoction
Food distention	TE1 太陰調胃湯 Taeeum Stomach-Regulating Decoction Fire : TE15 淸心蓮子湯	SE24 十二味寬中湯 Twelve-Flavor Middle-Soothing Decoction SE22 香砂養胃湯 Cyperi Rhizoma and	SY13 牧丹地黃湯 Moutan Cortex and Rehmanniae Radix Preparata Decoction SY45 李氏肥兒丸

	Heart-Clearing Nelumbinis Semen Decoction	Amomi Fructus Stomach-Nourishing Decoction Worse : ◆ 人蔘附子理中湯 Ginseng Radix and Aconiti Lateralis Radix Preparata Middle- Regulating Decoction	Lee's Child-Plumping Pill SY8 獨活地黃湯 Angelicae Pubescentis Radix and Rehmanniae Radix Preparata Decoction
Tympanites	TE15 清心蓮子湯 Heart-Clearing Nelumbinis Semen Decoction TE17 麻黃定痛湯 Ephedrae Herba Pain-Stabilizing Decoction	SE39 芎歸葱蘇理中湯 Cnidii, Angelicae Gigantis, Allii Fistulosi, and Perillae Middle- Regulating Decoction SE71 保命飮 Life-Protecting Decoction Stagnation: SE22 香砂養胃湯 Cyperi Rhizoma and Amomi Fructus Stomach-Nourishing Decoction SE24 十二味寬中湯 Twelve-Flavor Middle-Soothing Decoction	SY21 忍冬藤地骨皮湯 Lonicerae Caulis and Lycii Radicis Cortex Decoction

14) Wasting-Thirst

Symptom	Taeeum type	Soeum type	Soyang type
Upper wasting-thirst	TE58 萬金文武湯 Ten Thousand Gold Pieces Gentle-Firm Decoction	SE6 補中益氣湯 Middle-Tonifying Qi-Replenishing Decoction SE28 薑朮寬中湯 Zingiberis Rhizoma and Atractylodis Rhizoma Alba Middle-Soothing Decoction SE13 八物君子湯 Eight-Element Noble Decoction	SY20 凉膈散火湯 Diaphragm-Cooling Fire-Dissipating Decoction
Middle wasting-thirst	TE12 調胃升淸湯 Stomach-Regulating Upraising-Clearing Decoction TE19 清肺瀉肝湯 Lung-Clearing Liver-Purging Decoction	SE39 芎歸葱蘇理中湯 Cnidii, Angelicae Gigantis, Allii Fistulosi, and Perillae Middle-Regulating Decoction	SY21 忍冬藤地骨皮湯 Lonicerae Caulis and Lycii Radicis Cortex Decoction

Lower wasting-thirst	TE19 淸肺瀉肝湯 Lung-Clearing Liver-Purging Decoction TE57 千金文武湯 Thousand Gold Pieces Gentle-Firm Decoction	SE6 補中益氣湯 Middle-Tonifying Qi-Replenishing Decoction SE28 薑朮寬中湯 Zingiberis Rhizoma and Atractylodis Rhizoma Alba Middle-Soothing Decoction SE13 八物君子湯 Eight-Element Noble Decoction	SY22 熟地黃苦蔘湯 Rehmanniae Radix Preparata and Sophorae Radix Decoction SY38 黃連猪肚湯 Coptidis Rhizoma and Pig Stomach Decoction

15) Jaundice

Symptom	Taeeum type	Soeum type	Soyang type
In general	TE1 太陰調胃湯 Taeeum Stomach-Regulating Decoction TE51 退黃飮 Sallowness-Repelling Decoction	SE22 香砂養胃湯 Cyperi Rhizoma and Amomi Fructus Stomach-Nourishing Decoction SE60 茵陳橘皮湯 Artemisiae Capillaris Herba and Citrus Unshius Pericarpium Decoction SE58 茵陳四逆湯 Artemisiae Capillaris Herba Four Counterflow Decoction SE59 茵陳附子湯 Artemisiae Capillaris Herba and Aconiti Lateralis Radix Preparata Decoction SE64 瘴疸丸 Miasmic Jaundice Decoction SE31 巴豆丹 Crotonis Semen Pellet	Consumptive disease: SY9 荊防地黃湯 Schizonepetae, Saposhnikoviae, and Rehmanniae Radix Preparata Decoction Heat: SY4 荊防瀉白散 Schizonepetae Spica and Saposhnikoviae Radix White-Draining Powder SY6 猪苓車前子湯 Polyporus and Plantaginis Semen Decoction

16) Malaria

Symptom	Taeeum type	Soeum type	Soyang type
Malaria	Cold: TE1 太陰調胃湯 Taeeum Stomach-Regulating Decoction	SE9 川芎桂枝湯 Cnidii Rhizoma and Cinnamomi Ramulus	SY1 荊防敗毒散 Schizonepetae Spica and Saposhnikoviae

Symptom	Taeeum type	Soeum type	Soyang type
	Heat: TE11 葛根解肌湯 Puerariae Radix Flesh-Resolving Decoction Long-lasting overexertion : TE1 太陰調胃湯 Taeeum Stomach-Regulating Decoction	Decoction Long-lasting overexertion : SE30 鷄蔘膏 Chicken and Ginseng Radix Paste.	Radix Toxin-Repelling Powder SY8 獨活地黃湯 Angelicae Pubescentis Radix and Rehmanniae Radix Preparata Decoction Interior heat: SY4 荊防瀉白散 Schizonepetae Spica and Saposhnikoviae
	Pregnant women : TE7 經驗調胃湯 Empirical Stomach-Regulating Decoction		Radix White-Draining Powder, SY18 地黃白虎湯 Rehmanniae Radix Crudus White Tiger Powder

17) Mental Derangement

Symptom	Taeeum type	Soeum type	Soyang type
In general	TE-e16 四時丹 Four Seasons Pellet	SE63 溫白元 White-Warming Pill SE68 如意丹 Pliant Pellet	SY-e22 贊化丹 Transformation-Helping Pellet

18) Essense

Symptom	Taeeum type	Soeum type	Soyang type
Dream emission	TE15 淸心蓮子湯 Heart-Clearing Nelumbinis Semen Decoction TE19 淸肺瀉肝湯 Lung-Clearing Liver-Purging Decoction TE38 乾栗樗根皮湯 Castaneae Semen and Ailanthi Cortex Decoction TE20 定神瀉肝湯	SE6 補中益氣湯 Middle-Tonifying Qi-Replenishing Decoction ◆ 李氏補中益氣湯 Lee's Middle-Tonifying Qi-Replenishing Decoction ◆ 白朮散 或單服 Atractylodis Rhizoma Alba Powder or Atractylodis Rhizoma Alba only	SY41 六味地黃湯 Six-Element Rehmanniae Radix Preparata Decoction Steaming bone: SY17 十二味地黃湯 Twelve-Flavor Rehmanniae Radix Preparata Decoction

Symptom	Taeeum type	Soeum type	Soyang type
	Spirit-Stabilizing Liver-Purging Decoction		
White ooze	TE15 淸心蓮子湯 Heart-Clearing Nelumbinis Semen Decoction TE19 淸肺瀉肝湯 Lung-Clearing Liver-Purging Decoction	SE6 補中益氣湯 Middle-Tonifying Qi-Replenishing Decoction ◆ 李氏補中益氣湯 Lee's Middle-Tonifying Qi-Replenishing Decoction	SY41 六味地黃湯 Six-Element Rehmanniae Radix Preparata Decoction Steaming bone: SY17 十二味地黃湯 Twelve-Flavor Rehmanniae Radix Preparata Decoction
	TE20 定神瀉肝湯 Spirit-Stabilizing Liver-Purging Decoction TE38 乾栗樗根皮湯 Castaneae Semen and Holotrichia Decoction	白朮散 或單服 Atractylodis Rhizoma Alba Powder or Atractylodis Rhizoma Alba only	

19) Qi

Symptom	Taeeum type	Soeum type	Soyang type
Seven qi	TE15 淸心蓮子湯 Heart-Clearing Nelumbinis Semen Decoction TE41 麝香散 Moschus Powder	SE85 七氣湯 Seven Qi Decoction SE24 十二味寬中湯 加 五靈脂, 枳殼 Twelve-Flavor Middle-Soothing Decoction added Trogopterorum Faeces 五靈脂, Aurantii Fructus Immaturus 枳殼	SY20 凉膈散火湯 Diaphragm-Cooling Fire-Dissipating Decoction added Coptidis Rhizoma 黃連 and Arctii Fructus 牛蒡子
Qi depression	TE15 淸心蓮子湯 Heart-Clearing Nelumbinis Semen Decoction TE41 麝香散 Moschus Powder	SE86 正氣天香湯 Qi-Correcting Linderae Radix and Cyperi Rhizoma Decoction SE45 寬中丸 Middle-Soothing Pill	SY20 凉膈散火湯 Diaphragm-Cooling Fire-Dissipating Decoction
Nine qi	TE15 淸心蓮子湯 Heart-Clearing Nelumbinis Semen Decoction	SE86 正氣天香湯 Qi-Correcting Linderae Radix and Cyperi Rhizoma Decoction	SY20 凉膈散火湯 Diaphragm-Cooling Fire-Dissipating Decoction

Symptom	Taeeum type	Soeum type	Soyang type
	TE41 麝香散 Moschus Powder		
Qi stroke	TE42 石菖蒲遠志散 Acori Graminei Rhizoma and Polygalae Radix Powder TE55 滾痰湯 Phlegm-Sluicing Decoction	SE54 木香順氣散 Aucklandiae Radix Qi-Arranging Powder SE55 蘇合香元 Styrax Liquides Pill	SY26 朱砂益元散 Cinnabaris Prime-Replenishing Powder
Shortness of breath	TE1 太陰調胃湯 Taeeum Stomach-Regulating Decoction TE32 鹿茸大補湯 Cervi Parvum Cornu Greatly Tonifying Decoction TE31 拱辰黑元丹 Polaris-Aspiring Black Vitality Pellet ◆ 葛茸大補湯 Puerariae Surculus Greatly Tonifying Decoction	SE6 補中益氣湯 Middle-Tonifying Qi-Replenishing Decoction SE5 升陽益氣湯 Yang-Upraising Qi-Replenishing Decoction SE13 八物君子湯 Eight-Element Noble Decoction	SY41 六味地黃湯 Six-Element Rehmanniae Radix Preparata Decoction SY9 荊防地黃湯 Schizonepetae, Saposhnikoviae, and Rehmanniae Radix Preparata Decoction
Qi stagnation	TE42 石菖蒲遠志散 Acori Graminei Rhizoma and Polygalae Radix Powder TE55 滾痰湯 Phlegm-Sluicing Decoction	SE45 寬中湯 Middle-Soothing Decoction ◆ 橘皮一物湯 Citrus Unshius Pericarpium Single-Element Decoction	SY13 牧丹皮地黃湯 Moutan Cortex and Rehmanniae Radix Preparata Decoction
Qi pain	TE19 清肺瀉肝湯 Lung-Clearing Liver-Purging Decoction	SE45 寬中湯 Middle-Soothing Decoction ◆ 橘皮一物湯 Citrus Unshius Pericarpium Alone Decoction	SY13 牧丹皮地黃湯 Moutan Cortex and Rehmanniae Radix Preparata Decoction

20) Spirit

Symptom	Taeeum type	Soeum type	Soyang type
Fright palpitations	TE45 牛黃淸心元 Bovis Calculus Heart-Clearing Pill TE43 三神散 Three Spirit Powder	SE55 蘇合香元 Styrax Liquides Pill SE13 八物君子湯 Eight-Element Noble Decoction	SY41 六味地黃湯 Six-Element Rehmanniae Radix Preparata Decoction SY17 十二味地黃湯 Twelve-Flavor Rehmanniae Radix Preparata Decoction
Fearful throbbing	TE45 牛黃淸心元 Bovis Calculus Heart-Clearing Pill TE43 三神散 Three Spirit Powder	SE23 赤白何烏寬中湯 Polygoni Multiflori Radix and Cynanchi Wilfordii Radix Middle-Soothing Decoction	朱砂散 Cinnabaris Powder
Forgetfulness	TE43 三神散 Three Spirit Powder TE12 調胃升淸湯 Stomach-Regulating Upraising-Clearing Decoction	SE13 八物君子湯 Eight-Element Noble Decoction SE15 十全大補湯 Ten Wholesome Greatly Tonifying Decoction	SY41 六味地黃湯 Six-Element Rehmanniae Radix Preparata Decoction SY9 荊防地黃湯 Schizonepetae, Saposhnikoviae, and Rehmanniae Radix Preparata Decoction
Epilepsy	Heat: TE19 淸肺瀉肝湯 Lung-Clearing Liver-Purging Decoction Cold: TE45 牛黃淸心元 Bovis Calculus Heart-Clearing Pill TE42 石菖蒲遠志散 Acori Graminei Rhizoma and Polygalae Radix Powder TE43 三神散 Three Spirit Powder	SE16 獨蔘八物湯 Ginseng-Emphasized Eight-Element Decoction SE25 人蔘白何烏寬中湯 Ginseng Radix and Cynanchi Wilfordii Radix Middle-Soothing Decoction SE68 如意丹 Pliant Pellet	Heat: SY18 地黃白虎湯 Rehmanniae Radix Crudus White Tiger Decoction, SY17 十二味地黃湯 Twelve-Flavor Rehmanniae Radix Preparata Decoction Deficiency: SY9 荊防地黃湯 Schizonepetae, Saposhnikoviae, and Rehmanniae Radix Preparata Decoction
Depressive and manic psychosis	TE19 淸肺瀉肝湯 Lung-Clearing Liver-Purging Decoction TE45 牛黃淸心元	SE16 獨蔘八物湯 Ginseng-Emphasized Eight-Element Decoction SE25 人蔘白何烏寬中湯	Heat: SY18 地黃白虎湯 Rehmanniae Radix Crudus White Tiger Decoction, SY17 十二味地黃湯

Symptom	Taeeum type	Soeum type	Soyang type
	Bovis Calculus Heart-Clearing Pill TE42 石菖蒲遠志散 Acori Graminei Rhizoma and Polygalae Radix Powder TE43 三神散 Three Spirit Powder	Ginseng Radix and Cynanchi Wilfordii Radix Middle-Soothing Decoction SE68 如意丹 Pliant Pellet	Twelve-Flavor Rehmanniae Radix Preparata Decoction Deficiency: SY9 荊防地黃湯 Schizonepetae, Saposhnikoviae, and Rehmanniae Radix Preparata Decoction

21) Blood

Symptom	Taeeum type	Soeum type	Soyang type
Epistaxis	TE29 補肺元湯 Lung-Prime Tonifying Decoction	SE18 香附子八物湯 Cyperi Rhizoma Eight-Element Decoction	Deficiency: SY15 生熟地黃湯 Rehmanniae Radix Crudus et Preparata Decoction Fire: SY20 凉膈散火湯 Diaphragm-Cooling Fire-Dissipating Decoction
Hematemesis	TE15 淸心蓮子湯 Heart-Clearing Nelumbinis Semen Decoction Heat: TE19 淸肺瀉肝湯 Lung-Clearing Liver-Purging Decoction Overexertion: TE30 山藥補肺元湯 Dioscoreae Rhizoma Lung-Prime Tonifying Decoction added Nelumbinis Semen 蓮肉	SE16 獨蔘八物湯 Ginseng-Emphasized Eight-Element Decoction SE70 鎭陰膾 Yin-Suppressing Tartare SE15 十全大補湯 Ten Wholesome Greatly Tonifying Decoction SE6 補中益氣湯 Middle-Tonifying Qi-Replenishing Decoction	SY8 獨活地黃湯 Angelicae Pubescentis Radix and Rehmanniae Radix Preparata Decoction SY17 十二味地黃湯 Twelve-Flavor Rehmanniae Radix Preparata Decoction SY9 荊防地黃湯 Schizonepetae, Saposhnikoviae, and Rehmanniae Radix Preparata Decoction
Hematuria	TE19 淸肺瀉肝湯 Lung-Clearing Liver-Purging Decoction Sexual overindulgence: TE15 淸心蓮子湯 Heart- Clearing Nelumbinis Semen Decoction	SE23 赤白何烏寬中湯 Polygoni Multiflori Radix and Cynanchi Wilfordii Radix Middle-Soothing Decoction	SY15 生熟地黃湯 Rehmanniae Radix Crudus et Preparata Decoction SY20 凉膈散火湯 Diaphragm-Cooling Fire- Dissipating Decoction

Symptom	Taeeum type	Soeum type	Soyang type
Hematochezia	TE19 淸肺瀉肝湯 Lung-Clearing Liver-Purging Decoction TE15 淸心蓮子湯 Heart-Clearing Nelumbinis Semen Decoction	SE15 十全大補湯 Ten Wholesome Greatly Tonifying Decoction SE47 理中湯 Middle-Regulating Decoction SE22 香砂養胃湯 Cyperi Rhizoma and Amomi Fructus Stomach- Nourishing Decoction	SY20 涼膈散火湯 Diaphragm-Cooling Fire-Dissipating Decoction SY15 生熟地黃湯 Rehmanniae Radix Crudus et Preparata Decoction
Gum and tongue bleeding	TE24 葛根承氣湯 Puerariae Radix Qi-Coordinating Decoction	SE40 吳茱萸附子理中湯 Evodiae Fructus and Aconiti Lateralis Radix Preparata Middle- Regulating Decoction Blood sweating: SE6 補中益氣湯 Middle- Tonifying Qi-Replenishing Decoction SE3 升陽益氣附子湯 Yang-Upraising Qi-Replenishing Aconiti Lateralis Radix Preparata Decoction Bleeding from nine orifices: SE15 十全大補湯 Ten Wholesome Greatly Tonifying Decoction	SY19 陽毒白虎湯 Yang Toxin White Tiger Decoction SY51 催生散 Delivery-Inducing Powder
Vertigo due to blood loss	TE1 太陰調胃湯 Taeeum Stomach-Regulating Decoction TE30 山藥補肺元湯 Dioscoreae Rhizoma Lung-Prime Tonifying Decoction	SE13 八物君子湯 Eight-Element Noble Decoction SE6 補中益氣湯 Middle-Tonifying Qi-Replenishing Decoction SE5 升陽益氣湯 Yang-Upraising Qi-Replenishing Decoction	SY41 六味地黃湯 Six-Element Rehmanniae Radix Preparata Decoction SY8 獨活地黃湯 Angelicae Pubescentis Radix and Rehmanniae Radix Preparata Decoction

22) Voice

Symptom	Taeeum type	Soeum type	Soyang type
Loss of voice due to wind and cold	TE1 太陰調胃湯 Taeeum Stomach-Regulating Decoction TE44 麥門冬遠志散 Liriopis Tuber and Polygalae Radix Powder	SE9 川芎桂枝湯 Cnidii Rhizoma and Cinnamomi Ramulus Decoction ◆ 何烏八物湯 Polygoni Multiflori Radix Eight-Element Decoction	SY1 荊防敗毒散 Schizonepetae Spica and Saposhnikoviae Radix Toxin-Repelling Powder SY54 歸腎解語湯 Kidney-Restoring Speech- Releasing Decoction
Loss of voice due to sex indulgence damage	TE10 腎氣調胃湯 Kidney Qi Stomach-Regulating Decoction	SE15 十全大補湯 Ten Wholesome Greatly Tonifying Decoction SE6 補中益氣湯 Middle-Tonifying Qi-Replenishing Decoction	SY9 荊防地黃湯 Schizonepetae, Saposhnikoviae, and Rehmanniae Radix Preparata Decoction
Loss of voice during the convalescence of disease	TE27 調理肺元湯 Lung-Prime Regulating Decoction added Acori Graminei Rhizoma 石菖蒲	SE15 十全大補湯 Ten Wholesome Greatly Tonifying Decoction	◆ 六味腎氣湯 Six-Element Kidney Qi Decoction
Loss of voice due to wind stroke	TE56 祛風解語散 Wind-Dispelling Speech-Releasing Powder	SE84 壽脾解語湯 Spleen-Longevity Speech-Releasing Decoction SE21 祛風散 Wind-Dispelling Powder	SY54 歸腎解語湯 Kidney-Restoring Speech-Releasing Decoction
Loss of voice after childbirth	TE27 調理肺元湯 Lung-Prime Regulating Decoction TE29 補肺元湯 Lung-Prime Tonifying Decoction added Acori Graminei Rhizoma 石菖蒲	SE15 十全大補湯 Ten Wholesome Greatly Tonifying Decoction	SY9 荊防地黃湯 Schizonepetae, Saposhnikoviae, and Rehmanniae Radix Preparata Decoction SY1 荊防敗毒散 Schizonepetae Spica and Saposhnikoviae Radix Toxin-Repelling Powder

23) Fluid and humor

Symptom	Taeeum type	Soeum type	Soyang type
Spontaneous sweating and night sweating	TE12 調胃升淸湯 Stomach-Regulating Upraising-Clearing Decoction	SE6 補中益氣湯 Middle-Tonifying Qi-Replenishing Decoction	Upper wasting-thirst: SY39 凉膈散 Diaphragm-Cooling Powder Steaming bone : SY17 十二味地黃湯
			Twelve-Flavor Rehmanniae Radix Preparata Decoction, SY8 獨活地黃湯 Angelicae Pubescentis Radix and Rehmanniae Radix Preparata Decoction

24) Phlegm-Retained Fluid

Symptom	Taeeum type	Soeum type	Soyang type
Wind phlegm	TE9 調胃續命湯 Stomach-Regulating Life-Prolonging Decoction	SE21 祛風散 Wind-Dispelling Powder	SY1 荊防敗毒散 Schizonepetae Spica and Saposhnikoviae Radix Toxin-Repelling Powder
Cold phlegm	◆ 菖蒲透邪煎 Acori Graminei Rhizoma Pathogen-Outthrusting Decoction TE9 調胃續命湯 Stomach-Regulating Life-Prolonging Decoction TE40 熊膽散 Fel Ursi Powder	SE23 赤白何烏寬中湯 Polygoni Multiflori Radix and Cynanchi Wilfordii Radix Middle-Soothing Decoction SE47 理中湯 Middle-Regulating Decoction	SY1 荊防敗毒散 Schizonepetae Spica and Saposhnikoviae Radix Toxin-Repelling Powder
Dampness phlegm	◆ 菖蒲透邪煎 Acori Graminei Rhizoma Pathogen-Outthrusting Decoction TE9 調胃續命湯 Stomach-Regulating	SE23 赤白何烏寬中湯 Polygoni Multiflori Radix and Cynanchi Wilfordii Radix Middle-Soothing Decoction	SY4 荊防瀉白散 Schizonepetae Spica and Saposhnikoviae Radix White-Draining Powder

Symptom	Taeeum type	Soeum type	Soyang type
	Life-Prolonging Decoction TE40 熊膽散 Fel Ursi Powder		
Heat phlegm	TE19 淸肺瀉肝湯 Lung-Clearing Liver-Purging Decoction	SE25 人蔘白何烏寬中湯 Ginseng Radix and Cynanchi Wilfordii Radix Middle-Soothing Decoction SE6 補中益氣湯 Middle-Tonifying Qi-Replenishing Decoction SE26 當歸白何烏寬中湯 Angelicae Gigantis Radix and Polygoni Multiflori Radix Alba Middle-Soothing Decoction	SY20 凉膈散火湯 Diaphragm-Cooling Fire-Dissipating Decoction SY19 陽毒白虎湯 Yang Toxin White Tiger Decoction
Stagnated phlegm	TE19 淸肺瀉肝湯 Lung-Clearing Liver-Purging Decoction	SE26 當歸白何烏寬中湯 Angelicae Gigantis Radix and Polygoni Multiflori Radix Alba Middle-Soothing Decoction	SY20 凉膈散火湯 Diaphragm-Cooling Fire-Dissipating Decoction
Qi phlegm	TE55 滾痰湯 Phlegm-Sluicing Decoction	SE45 寬中湯 Middle-Soothing Decoction	導赤降氣湯 Red-Conducting Qi-Lowering Decoction
Food phlegm	TE1 太陰調胃湯 Taeeum Stomach-Regulating Decoction	SE22 香砂養胃湯 Cyperi Rhizoma and Amomi Fructus Stomach-Nourishing Decoction	SY41 六味地黃湯 Six-Element Rehmanniae Radix Preparata Decoction
Alcoholic phlegm	TE18 熱多寒少湯 Heat-Dominant Cold-Recessive Decoction	SE92 星香正氣散 Arisaematis Rhizoma and Aucklandiae Radix Qi-Correcting Powder	SY40 李氏凉膈散 Lee's Diaphragm-Cooling Powder SY4 荊防瀉白散 Schizonepetae Spica and Saposhnikoviae Radix White-Draining Powder
Phlegm induced by fright	TE55 滾痰湯 Phlegm-Sluicing	SE55 蘇合香元 Styrax Liquides Pill	SY26 朱砂益元散 Cinnabaris

Symptom	Taeeum type	Soeum type	Soyang type
	Decoction TE42 石菖蒲遠志散 Acori Graminei Rhizoma and Polygalae Radix Powder	SE63 溫白元 White-Warming Pill	Prime-Replenishing Powder
Running phlegm	TE19 淸肺瀉肝湯 Lung-Clearing Liver-Purging Decoction	SE24 十二味寬中湯 Twelve-Flavor Middle-Soothing Decoction SE21 祛風散 Wind-Dispelling Powder	SY19 陽毒白虎湯 Yang Toxin White Tiger Decoction SY31 輕粉乳香沒藥丸 Calomelas, Olibanum, and Myrrha Pill
Phlegm syncope	Cold: ◆ 菖蒲透邪煎 Acori Graminei Rhizoma Pathogen-Outthrusting Decoction Heat: TE24 葛根承氣湯 Puerariae Radix Qi-Coordinating Decoction	SE92 星香正氣散 Arisaematis Rhizoma and Aucklandiae Radix Qi-Correcting Powder	SE5 黃連導白散 Coptidis Rhizoma White-Conducting Powder
Phlegm mass	TE19 淸肺瀉肝湯 Lung-Clearing Liver-Purging Decoction	SE63 溫白元 White-Warming Pill SE24 十二味寬中湯 Twelve-Flavor Middle-Soothing Decoction SE39 芎歸葱蘇理中湯 Cnidii, Angelicae Gigantis, Allii Fistulosi, and Perillae Middle-Regulating Decoction	SY19 陽毒白虎湯 Yang Toxin White Tiger Decoction SY31 輕粉乳香沒藥丸 Calomelas, Olibanum, and Myrrha Pill

25) Worm

Symptom	Taeeum type	Soeum type	Soyang type
Ascaris (syncope)	TE17 麻黃定痛湯 Ephedrae Herba Pain-Stabilizing Decoction	SE43 白何烏理中湯 Cynanchi Wilfordii Radix Middle-Regulating Decoction SE42 白何烏附子理中湯	SY7 滑石苦蔘湯 Talcum and Sophorae Radix Decoction SY41 六味地黃湯 Six-Element

		Cynanchi Wilfordii Radix and Aconiti Lateralis Radix Preparata Middle-Regulating Decoction	Rehmanniae Radix Preparata Decoction

26) Urine

Symptom	Taeeum type	Soeum type	Soyang type
Inhibited urination	Deficiency: TE1 太陰調胃湯 Taeeum Stomach-Regulating Decoction Heat: TE18 熱多寒少湯 Heat-Dominant Cold-Recessive Decoction	SE23 赤白何烏寬中湯 Polygoni Multiflori Radix and Cynanchi Wilfordii Radix Middle-Soothing Decoction Deficiency: ◆ 李氏補中益氣湯 Lee's Middle-Tonifying Qi-Replenishing Decoction	SY6 猪苓車前子湯 Polyporus and Plantaginis Semen Decoction Deficiency: SY16 木通無憂湯 Akebiae Caulis Anxiety-Free Decoction Excess heat: SY18 地黃白虎湯 Rehmanniae Radix Crudus White Tiger Decoction
Urinary incontinence	It should be treated according to the treatments of three wasting.	SE6 補中益氣湯 Middle-Tonifying Qi-Replenishing Decoction SE47 理中湯 Middle-Regulating Decoction	SY41 六味地黃湯 Six-Element Rehmanniae Radix Preparata Decoction SY20 凉膈散火湯 Diaphragm-Cooling Fire-Dissipating Decoction
Five types of stranguria	Cold: TE1 太陰調胃湯 Taeeum Stomach-Regulating Decoction Heat: TE18 熱多寒少湯 Heat-Dominant Cold-Recessive Decoction	SE28 薑朮寬中湯 Zingiberis Rhizoma and Atractylodis Rhizoma Alba Middle-Soothing Decoction SE6 補中益氣湯 Middle-Tonifying Qi-Replenishing Decoction added Cyperi Rhizoma 香附 and Cnidii Rhizoma 川芎	SY9 荊防地黃湯 Schizonepetae, Saposhnikoviae, and Rehmanniae Radix Preparata Decoction SY25 荊芥清腸湯 Schizonepetae Spica Intestine-Cooling Decoction SY6 猪苓車前子湯 Polyporus and Plantaginis Semen Decoction added Akebiae Caulis 木通 and Rehmanniae Radix Crudus 生地黃

Symptom	Taeeum type	Soeum type	Soyang type
Itching and pain in the penis	TE15 淸心蓮子湯 Heart-Clearing Nelumbinis Semen Decoction TE18 熱多寒少湯 Heat-Dominant Cold-Recessive Decoction	SE28 薑朮寬中湯 Zingiberis Rhizoma and Atractylodis Rhizoma Alba Middle-Soothing Decoction SE6 補中益氣湯 Middle-Tonifying Qi-Replenishing Decoction added Cyperi Rhizoma 香附 and Cnidii Rhizoma 川芎	SY3 導赤降氣湯 Red-Conducting Qi-Lowering Decoction
Recto-urethral fistula	TE1 太陰調胃湯 Taeeum Stomach-Regulating Decoction TE18 熱多寒少湯 Heat-Dominant Cold-Recessive Decoction	SE6 補中益氣湯 Middle-Tonifying Qi-Replenishing Decoction SE13 八物君子湯 Eight-Element Noble Decoction	SY6 猪苓車前子湯 Polyporus and Plantaginis Semen Decoction SY9 荊防地黃湯 Schizonepetae, Saposhnikoviae, and Rehmanniae Radix Preparata Decoction

27) Stool

Symptom	Taeeum type	Soeum type	Soyang type
Dietary diarrhea	TE1 太陰調胃湯 Taeeum Stomach-Regulating Decoction TE15 淸心蓮子湯 Heart-Clearing Nelumbinis Semen Decoction	SE22 香砂養胃湯 Cyperi Rhizoma and Amomi Fructus Stomach-Nourishing Decoction SE91 藿香正氣散 Agastachis Herba Qi-Correcting Powder SE42 白何烏附子理中湯 Cynanchi Wilfordii Radix and Aconiti Lateralis Radix Preparata Middle-Regulating Decoction	SY13 牧丹皮地黃湯 Moutan Cortex and Rehmanniae Radix Preparata Decoction SY-e22 贊化丹 Transformation-Helping Pellet
Summerheat diarrhea	TE11 葛根解肌湯 Puerariae Radix Flesh-Resolving Decoction	SE43 白何烏理中湯 Cynanchi Wilfordii Radix Middle-Regulating Decoction	SY26 朱砂益元散 Cinnabaris Prime-Replenishing Powder

Symptom	Taeeum type	Soeum type	Soyang type
	◆ 李氏調胃湯 Lee's Stomach-Regulating Decoction	SE42 白何烏附子理中湯 Cynanchi Wilfordii Radix and Aconiti Lateralis Radix Preparata Middle-Regulating Decoction	SY6 猪苓車前子湯 Polyporus and Plantaginis Semen Decoction
Deficiency diarrhea	TE1 太陰調胃湯 Taeeum Stomach-Regulating Decoction TE15 淸心蓮子湯 Heart-Clearing Nelumbinis Semen Decoction	SE43 白何烏理中湯 Cynanchi Wilfordii Radix Middle-Regulating Decoction SE42 白何烏附子理中湯 Cynanchi Wilfordii Radix and Aconiti Lateralis Radix Preparata Middle-Regulating Decoction ◆ 人蔘附子理中湯 Ginseng Radix and Aconiti Lateralis Radix Preparata Middle-Regulating Decoction	SY13 牧丹皮地黃湯 Moutan Cortex and Rehmanniae Radix Preparata Decoction SY6 猪苓車前子湯 Polyporus and Plantaginis Semen Decoction
Kidney diarrhea	TE10 腎氣調胃湯 Kidney Qi Stomach-Regulating Decoction TE15 淸心蓮子湯 Heart-Clearing Nelumbinis Semen Decoction	◆ 人蔘附子理中湯 Ginseng Radix and Aconiti Lateralis Radix Preparata Middle-Regulating Decoction (Or use Cynanchi Wilfordii Radix 白何首烏 as sovereign medicinal, and double Atractylodis Rhizoma Alba 白朮)	SY16 木通無憂湯 Akebiae Caulis Anxiety-Free Decoction
Dysentery	TE38 乾栗樗根皮湯 Castaneae Semen and Holotrichia Decoction TE15 淸心蓮子湯 Heart-Clearing Nelumbinis Semen Decoction TE24 葛根承氣湯 Puerariae Radix Qi-Coordinating Decoction	SE22 香砂養胃湯 Cyperi Rhizoma and Amomi Fructus Stomach-Nourishing Decoction SE73 蒜蜜膏 Garlic and Honey Paste SE30 鷄蔘膏 Chicken and Ginseng Radix Paste SE72 赤蛇煎	◆ 黃連淸腸湯 Intestines clearing Decoction of Coptidis Rhizoma SY16 木通無憂湯 Akebiae Caulis Anxiety-Free Decoction

Symptom	Taeeum type	Soeum type	Soyang type
		Red-Colored Serpent Decoction (If there is a lot of cold, choose and use 理中湯 Middle-Regulationg Decoction)	
Constipation	TE24 葛根承氣湯 Puerariae Radix Qi-Coordinating Decoction ◆ 調胃承氣湯 Stomach-Regulating Qi-Coordinating Decoction Severe deficiency: TE59 二門五味湯 Liriope, Asparagus, and Schisandrae Decoction	SE31 巴豆丹 Crotonis Semen Pellet SE28 薑朮寬中湯 Zingiberis Rhizoma and Atractylodis Rhizoma Alba Middle-Soothing Decoction	SY18 地黃白虎湯 Rehmanniae Radix Crudus White Tiger Decoction SY28 輕粉甘隧龍虎丹 Calomelas and Euphorbiae Kansui Radix Dragon-Tiger Pellet

28) Head

Symptom	Taeeum type	Soeum type	Soyang type
Headache	Cold: TE1 太陰調胃湯 Taeeum Stomach-Regulating Decoction Heat: TE11 葛根解肌湯 Puerariae Radix Flesh-Resolving Decoction Wind: TE53 如神炷 Marvelous Incense Stick Phlegm: TE18 熱多寒少湯 Heat-Dominant Cold-Recessive Decoction Hemilateral headache : TE11 葛根解肌湯 Puerariae Radix Flesh-Resolving Decoction	SE6 補中益氣湯 Middle-Tonifying Qi-Replenishing Decoction SE13 八物君子湯 Eight-Element Noble Decoction Depression : SE18 香附子八物湯 Cyperi Rhizoma Eight-Element Decoction Wind-phlegm : SE21 祛風散 Wind-Dispelling Powder added Cnidii Rhizoma 川芎	SY9 荊防地黃湯 Schizonepetae, Saposhnikoviae, and Rehmanniae Radix Preparata Decoction Excess heat: SY18 地黃白虎湯 Rehmanniae Radix Crudus White Tiger Decoction Wind: SY1 荊防敗毒散 Schizonepetae Spica and Saposhnikoviae Radix Toxin-Repelling Powder Phlegm: SY3 導赤降氣湯 Red-Conducting Qi-Lowering Decoction SY20 凉膈散火湯 Diaphragm-Cooling Fire-Dissipating Decoction Hemilateral headache: SY12 黃連地黃湯 Coptidis Rhizoma and Rehmanniae Radix Preparata Decoction

29) Face

Symptom	Taeeum type	Soeum type	Soyang type
Facial heat	TE18 熱多寒少湯 Heat-Dominant Cold-Recessive Decoction Sexual taxation : TE15 清心蓮子湯 Heart-Clearing Nelumbinis Semen Decoction	SE6 補中益氣湯 Middle-Tonifying Qi-Replenishing Decoction	SY20 凉膈散火湯 Diaphragm-Cooling Fire-Dissipating Decoction Steaming bone: SY17 十二味地黃湯 Twelve-Flavor Rehmanniae Radix Preparata Decoction
Facial coldness	TE1 太陰調胃湯 Taeeum Stomach-Regulating Decoction Yellowish black: TE18 熱多寒少湯 Heat-Dominant Cold-Recessive Decoction	SE42 白何烏附子理中湯 Cynanchi Wilfordii Radix and Aconiti Lateralis Radix Preparata Middle-Regulating Decoction ◆ 人蔘附子理中湯 Ginseng Radix and Aconiti Lateralis Radix Preparata Middle-Regulating Decoction	SY9 荊防地黃湯 Schizonepetae, Saposhnikoviae, and Rehmanniae Radix Preparata Decoction SY17 十二味地黃湯 Twelve-Flavor Rehmanniae Radix Preparata Decoction
Wind heat	TE18 熱多寒少湯 Heat-Dominant Cold-Recessive Decoction	SE13 八物君子湯 Eight-Element Noble Decoction	SY20 凉膈散火湯 Diaphragm-Cooling Fire-Dissipating Decoction
Freckle	◆ Pound Angelicae Tenuissimae Radix 藁本, Dried Castaneae Semen 黃栗, Angelicae Dahuricae Radix 白芷. And wash a face with them. ◆ 西施玉容散 Xi Shi's Beautiful Face Powder (can also be used for Soeum and Soyang types.)	◆ Pound Phaseoli Radiati Semen 綠豆, Agastachis Herba 藿香. And wash a face with them.	◆ Pound Phaseoli Saposhnikoviae Radix 防風, Trichosanthis Radix 天花粉. And wash a face with them.

30) Eyes

Symptom	Taeeum type	Soeum type	Soyang type
In general	Cold: TE1 太陰調胃湯 Taeeum Stomach-Regulating	SE6 補中益氣湯 Middle-Tonifying Qi-Replenishing	SY9 荊防地黃湯 Schizonepetae, Saposhnikoviae, and

Symptom	Taeeum type	Soeum type	Soyang type
	Decoction Heat: TE18 熱多寒少湯 Heat-Dominant Cold-Recessive Decoction	Decoction SE15 十全大補湯 Ten Wholesome Greatly Tonifying Decoction	Rehmanniae Radix Preparata Decoction SY15 生熟地黃湯 Rehmanniae Radix Crudus et Preparata Decoction
	Washing medicine: TE52 立效散 Immediate Effect Powder	SE13 八物君子湯 Eight-Element Noble Decoction Miscellaneous medicine : SE79 煖肝散 Liver-Warming Powder, SE80 硫黃散 Sulfur Powder	Fire: SY20 凉膈散火湯 Diaphragm-Cooling Fire-Dissipating Decoction, SY40 李氏凉膈散 Lee's Diaphragm-Cooling Powder Cold and heat: SY19 陽毒白虎湯 Yang Toxin White Tiger Decoction Miscellaneous medicine: SY50 點眼散 Eye Drop Powder (can also be used for Taeeum and Soeum types.)
Eye dropping	TE60 明目散 Eye-Brightening Powder (can also be used for Soeum and Soyang types.)		

31) Ear

Symptom	Taeeum type	Soeum type	Soyang type
Deafness	TE10 腎氣調胃湯 Kidney Qi Stomach-Regulating Decoction TE32 鹿茸大補湯 Cervi Parvum Cornu Greatly Tonifying Decoction ◆ 葛茸大補湯 Puerariae Surculus Greatly Tonifying Decoction	SE13 八物君子湯 Eight-Element Noble Decoction SE15 十全大補湯 Ten Wholesome Greatly Tonifying Decoction	SY9 荊防地黃湯 Schizonepetae, Saposhnikoviae, and Rehmanniae Radix Preparata Decoction
Tinnitus	TE10 腎氣調胃湯 Kidney Qi Stomach-Regulating Decoction	SE13 八物君子湯 Eight-Element Noble Decoction	SY9 荊防地黃湯 Schizonepetae, Saposhnikoviae, and Rehmanniae Radix Preparata Decoction
	TE32 鹿茸大補湯 Cervi Parvum Cornu	SE15 十全大補湯 Ten Wholesome Greatly	

Symptom	Taeeum type	Soeum type	Soyang type
	Greatly Tonifying Decoction ◆ 葛茸大補湯 Puerariae Surculus Greatly Tonifying Decoction	Tonifying Decoction	
Suppurative otitis media	TE11 葛根解肌湯 Puerariae Radix Flesh-Resolving Decoction	SE13 八物君子湯 Eight-Element Noble Decoction SE15 十全大補湯 Ten Wholesome Greatly Tonifying Decoction	SY20 凉膈散火湯 Diaphragm-Cooling Fire-Dissipating Decoction

32) Nose

Symptom	Taeeum type	Soeum type	Soyang type
Sinusitis	TE11 葛根解肌湯 Puerariae Radix Flesh-Resolving Decoction TE24 葛根承氣湯 Puerariae Radix Qi-Coordinating Decoction TE53 如神炷 Marvelous Incense Stick	SE15 十全大補湯 Ten Wholesome Greatly Tonifying Decoction	SY19 陽毒白虎湯 Yang Toxin White Tiger Decoction SY20 凉膈散火湯 Diaphragm-Cooling Fire-Dissipating Decoction
Nasal obstruction	TE53 如神炷 Marvelous Incense Stick	SE10 芎歸香蘇散 Cnidii, Angelicae Gigantis, Cyperi, and Perillae Powder added Asiasari Radix et Rhizoma 細辛 and Piperis Nigri Fructus 胡椒	SY1 荊防敗毒散 Schizonepetae Spica and Saposhnikoviae Radix Toxin-Repelling Powder
Nasal pain	None	◆ 李氏補中益氣湯 Lee's Middle-Tonifying Qi-Replenishing Decoction	None
Nasal polyp	TE19 淸肺瀉肝湯 Lung-Clearing Liver-Purging Decoction	SE15 十全大補湯 Ten Wholesome Greatly Tonifying Decoction	SY4 荊防瀉白散 Schizonepetae Spica and Saposhnikoviae Radix White-Draining Powder
Nasal sore	TE53 如神炷 Marvelous Incense Stick	SE13 八物君子湯 Eight-Element Noble Decoction	SY20 凉膈散火湯 Diaphragm-Cooling Fire-Dissipating Decoction

33) Mouth and Tongue

	Taeeum type	Soeum type	Soyang type
Mouth and Tongue	◆ 調中湯 Middle-Harmonizing Decoction TE47 黑奴丸 Black Ustilago Pill TE50 二聖救苦丸 Two Holy Suffering-Saving Pill (The above three prescriptions can contain TE60 Myeongmok-san 明目散 Eye-Brightening Powder.)	SE13 八物君子湯 Eight-Element Noble Decoction SE74 人蔘散 Ginseng Radix Powder	SY20 凉膈散火湯 Diaphragm-Cooling Fire-Dissipating Decoction SY19 陽毒白虎湯 Yang Toxin White Tiger Decoction SY45 李氏肥兒丸 Lee's Child-Plumping Pill Lip swelling[6] : SY47 水銀薰鼻方 Hydrargyrum Nose-Fumigating Formula SY31 輕粉乳香沒藥丸 Calomelas, Olibanum, and Myrrha Pill

34) Teeth

	Taeeum type	Soeum type	Soyang type
Teeth	TE53 如神炷 Marvelous Incense Stick TE54 歸腎一擦光 Kidney-Restoring Brightening Polish	SE6 補中益氣湯 Middle-Tonifying Qi-Replenishing Decoction SE21 祛風散 Wind-Dispelling Powder SE84 壽脾解語湯 Spleen-Longevity Speech-Releasing Decoction	SY1 荊防敗毒散 Schizonepetae Spica and Saposhnikoviae Radix Toxin-Repelling Powder SY20 凉膈散火湯 Diaphragm-Cooling Fire-Dissipating Decoction SY19 陽毒白虎湯 Yang Toxin White Tiger Decoction SY51 催生散 Delivery-Inducing Powder

6) This disease is more presented to Soyang type than other types.

35) Throat

Symptom	Taeeum type	Soeum type	Soyang type
Tonsillitis	TE18 熱多寒少湯 Heat-Dominant Cold-Recessive Decoction ◆ 大承氣湯 Major Qi-Coordinating Decoction TE53 如神炷 Marvelous Incense Stick Deficiency: TE1 太陰調胃湯 Taeeum Stomach-Regulating Decoction added Cimicifugae Rhizoma 升麻 and Angelicae Dahuricae Radix 白芷	SE72 赤蛇煎 Red-Colored Serpent Decoction SE16 獨蔘八物湯 Ginseng-Emphasized Eight-Element Decoction SE70 鎭陰膾 Yin-Suppressing Tartare SE63 溫白元 White-Warming Pill	SY20 涼膈散火湯 Diaphragm-Cooling Fire-Dissipating Decoction SY19 陽毒白虎湯 Yang Toxin White Tiger Decoction SY27 甘遂天一丸 Euphorbiae Kansui Radix Heaven-One Pill Severe and critical pattern : SY47 水銀薰鼻方 Hydrargyrum Nose-Fumigating Formula SY31 輕粉乳香沒藥丸 Calomelas, Olibanum, and Myrrha Pill
All symptoms	TE18 熱多寒少湯 Heat-Dominant Cold-Recessive Decoction TE53 如神炷 Marvelous Incense Stick	SE72 赤蛇煎 Red-Colored Serpent Decoction SE16 獨蔘八物湯 Ginseng-Emphasized Eight-Element Decoction	SY20 涼膈散火湯 Diaphragm-Cooling Fire-Dissipating Decoction SY27 甘遂天一丸 Euphorbiae Kansui Radix Heaven-One Pill
	Deficiency: TE1 太陰調胃湯 Taeeum Stomach-Regulating Decoction	SE70 鎭陰膾 Yin-Suppressing Tartare SE63 溫白元 White-Warming Pill	Severe and critical pattern : SY47 水銀薰鼻方 Hydrargyrum Nose-Fumigating Formula SY31 輕粉乳香沒藥丸 Calomelas, Olibanum, and Myrrha Pill Entwining-throat-wind[7] part is same as the lip-swelling one.
Mistakenly swallowed insects, bones, and steel etc.	TE59 二門五味湯 Liriope, Asparagus, and Schisandrae Decoction added Rhei Rhizoma	SE93 砂仁散 Amomi Fructus Powder or use Angelicae Gigantis	SY51 催生散Delivery-Inducing Powder or SY41 六味地黃湯

Symptom	Taeeum type	Soeum type	Soyang type
	大黃 and Cimicifugae Rhizoma 升麻 Pound Miribalite 朴硝, Talcum 滑石, Magnetitum 磁石 and take with lard 猪脂.	Radix 當歸 and Cnidii Rhizoma 川芎 Critical pattern : Decoct 112.5g of Ginseng Radix 人蔘, 18.75g of Angelicae Gigantis Radix 當歸, 18.75g of Cnidii Rhizoma 川芎 and 煎and mix with honey.	Six-Element Rehmanniae Radix Preparata Decoction

36) Chest

Symptom	Taeeum type	Soeum type	Soyang type
Chest pain	TE17 麻黃定痛湯 Ephedrae Herba Pain-Stabilizing Decoction	Same with cold-damage or chest bind part. Visceral bind: SE25 人蔘白何烏寬中湯 Ginseng Radix and Cynanchi Wilfordii Radix Middle- Soothing Decoction SE45 寬中湯 Middle-Soothing Decoction ◆ 人蔘附子理中湯 Ginseng Radix and Aconiti Lateralis Radix Preparata Middle-Regulating Decoction	Same with cold-damage or chest bind part.

37) Breast

Symptom	Taeeum type	Soeum type	Soyang type
Promote lactation	TE29 補肺元湯 Lung-Prime Tonifying Decoction	SE18 香附子八物湯 Cyperi Rhizoma Eight-Element Decoction	SY61 通乳歸腎湯 Lactation-Inducing Kidney-Restoring Decoction

7) A severe throat infection with redness entwining the fauces in the interior and swelling surrounding the neck at the exterior. (WHO-IST)

Symptom	Taeeum type	Soeum type	Soyang type
	TE61 補肺通乳散 Lung-Tonifying Lactation-Inducing Powder	SE56 香蘇散 Cyperi Rhizoma and Perillae Folium Powder SE87 甘橘煎 Citrus Unshiu Decoction	SY41 六味地黃湯 Six-Element Rehmanniae Radix Preparata Decoction
Acute mastitis	TE18 熱多寒少湯 Heat-Dominant Cold-Recessive Decoction Deficiency: TE9 調胃續命湯 Stomach-Regulating Life-Prolonging Decoction	SE13 八物君子湯 Eight-Element Noble Decoction SE15 十全大補湯 Ten Wholesome Greatly Tonifying Decoction	SY3 導赤降氣湯 Red-Conducting Qi-Lowering Decoction SY20 凉膈散火湯 Diaphragm-Cooling Fire-Dissipating Decoction
Stop lactation	Schisandrae Fructus 五味子, Nelumbinis Semen 蓮肉, etc.	Astragali Radix 黃芪, Ginseng Radix 人蔘, etc.	Rehmanniae Radix Preparata熟地黃 , Rehmanniae Radix Crudus 生地黃, etc.

38) Abdomen

Symptom	Taeeum type	Soeum type	Soyang type
Pain	TE15 淸心蓮子湯 Heart-Clearing Nelumbinis Semen Decoction TE1 太陰調胃湯 Taeeum Stomach- Regulating Decoction Acute pain : TE41 麝香散 Moschus Powder Flapping Abdomen Syndrome: TE1 太陰調胃湯 Taeeum Stomach-Regulating Decoction	SE47 理中湯 Middle-Regulating Decoction SE45 寬中湯 Middle-Soothing Decoction Flapping Abdomen Syndrome: SE47 理中湯 Middle-Regulating Decoction	SY9 荊防地黃湯 Schizonepetae, Saposhnikoviae, and Rehmanniae Radix Preparata Decoction SY7 滑石苦蔘湯 Talcum and Sophorae Radix Decoction Flapping Abdomen Syndrome: SY41 六味地黃湯 Six-Element Rehmanniae Radix Preparata Decoction

39) Waist

Symptom	Taeeum type	Soeum type	Soyang type
Lumbago	TE1 太陰調胃湯 Taeeum Stomach-Regulating Decoction ◆ 葛茸大補湯 Puerariae Surculus Greatly Tonifying Decoction	SE6 補中益氣湯 Middle-Tonifying Qi-Replenishing Decoction SE24 十二味寬中湯 Twelve-Flavor Middle-Soothing Decoction	SY9 荊防地黃湯 Schizonepetae, Saposhnikoviae, and Rehmanniae Radix Preparata Decoction SY41 六味地黃湯 Six-Element Rehmanniae Radix Preparata Decoction
Strain and contusion lumbago	TE56 三黃散 Three yellows Powder	SE88 如神湯 Marvelous Decoction	SY30 乳香沒藥輕粉丸 Myrrha, Olibanum, and Calomelas Pill

40) Hypochondrium

Same with the qi part. the left side belongs to qi, and the right side belongs to blood.

41) Skin

Symptom	Taeeum type	Soeum type	Soyang type
Urticaria	Same as the joint-running wind section.		
Itch and numbness	Same as the moving impediment and the hemiplegia section.	Same as the moving impediment and the hemiplegia section.	Same as the moving impediment and the hemiplegia section. Or add Coptidis Rhizoma 黃連 and Trichosanthis Semen 瓜蔞仁

42) Upper Limbs

Symptom	Taeeum type	Soeum type	Soyang type
Brachial pain	TE1 太陰調胃湯 Taeeum Stomach-Regulating Decoction TE18 熱多寒少湯 Heat-Dominant Cold-Recessive Decoction	SE9 川芎桂枝湯 Cnidii Rhizoma and Cinnamomi Ramulus Decoction SE24 十二味寬中湯 Twelve-Flavor Middle-Soothing Decoction	SY3 導赤降氣湯 Red-Conducting Qi-Lowering Decoction

43) Lower Limbs

Symptom	Taeeum type	Soeum type	Soyang type
In general	Deficiency: TE1 太陰調胃湯 Taeeum Stomach-Regulating Decoction Heat: TE19 淸肺瀉肝湯 Lung-Clearing Liver-Purging Decoction	SE13 八物君子湯 Eight-Element Noble Decoction added 7.5g of Atractylodis Rhizoma 蒼朮 and 7.5g of Cynanchi Wilfordii Radix 白何首烏	Fire: SY20 凉膈散火湯 Diaphragm-Cooling Fire-Dissipating Decoction Dampness: SY3 導赤降氣湯 Red-Conducting Qi-Lowering Decoction Wind: SY1 荊防敗毒散 Schizonepetae Spica and Saposhnikoviae Radix Toxin-Repelling Powder
			Deficiency with Wind-Dampness : SY8 獨活地黃湯 Angelicae Pubescentis Radix and Rehmanniae Radix Preparata Decoction Crane's knee Wind: SY9 荊防地黃湯 Schizonepetae, Saposhnikoviae, and Rehmanniae Radix Preparata Decoction

44) Anterior Yin

Symptom	Taeeum type	Soeum type	Soyang type
Abdominal colic	Deficiency: TE5 升芷調胃湯 Cimicifugae Rhizoma and Angelicae Dahuricae Radix Stomach-Regulating Decoction Heat: TE18 熱多寒少湯 Heat-Dominant Cold-Recessive Decoction	SE6 補中益氣湯 Middle-Tonifying Qi-Replenishing Decoction Severe cold: SE47 理中湯 Middle-Regulating Decoction	SY17 十二味地黃湯 Twelve-Flavor Rehmanniae Radix Preparata Decoction SY9 荊防地黃湯 Schizonepetae, Saposhnikoviae, and Rehmanniae Radix Preparata Decoction
Swelling of the scrotum	Deficiency: TE1 太陰調胃湯 Taeeum	SE6 補中益氣湯 Middle-Tonifying	SY17 十二味地黃湯 Twelve-Flavor

Symptom	Taeeum type	Soeum type	Soyang type
	Stomach-Regulating Decoction Heat: TE18 熱多寒少湯 Heat-Dominant Cold-Recessive Decoction	Qi-Replenishing Decoction Severe cold: SE47 理中湯 Middle-Regulating Decoction	Rehmanniae Radix Preparata Decoction SY9 荊防地黃湯 Schizonepetae, Saposhnikoviae, and Rehmanniae Radix Preparata Decoction
Yin collapse	TE2 花惜調胃湯 Piteous Flower Stomach-Regulating Decoction added Fossilia Ossis Mastodi 龍骨, Asini Corii Colla 阿膠 and Cervi Cornus Colla 鹿角膠 should be substituted for Leiocassis Longirostris 民魚.	SE11 秘傳香蘇散 Secret Cyperi Rhizoma and Perillae Folium Powder SE7 九味花惜湯 Nine-Flavor Piteous Flower Decoction	SY42 花惜地黃湯 Piteous Flower Rehmanniae Radix Preparata Decoction
Pudendal swelling and itch	The prescription is the same as for the abdominal colic section. Steam, partake or wash.		

45) Posterior Yin

Symptom	Taeeum type	Soeum type	Soyang type
Hemorrhoidal fistula	TE1 太陰調胃湯 Taeeum Stomach-Regulating Decoction	SE6 補中益氣湯 Middle-Tonifying Qi-Replenishing Decoction SE15 十全大補湯 Ten Wholesome Greatly Tonifying Decoction	SY1 荊防敗毒散 Schizonepetae Spica and Saposhnikoviae Radix Toxin-Repelling Powder SY41 六味地黃湯 Six-Element Rehmanniae Radix Preparata Decoction Heat toxin: SE5 黃連導白散 Coptidis Rhizoma White-Conducting Powder

46) Abscess and Carbuncle

Symptom	Taeeum type	Soeum type	Soyang type
Early stage	TE11 葛根解肌湯 Puerariae Radix	SE9 川芎桂枝湯 Cnidii Rhizoma and	SY46 消毒飮 Toxin-Dissolving

Symptom	Taeeum type	Soeum type	Soyang type
	Flesh-Resolving Decoction	Cinnamomi Ramulus Decoction SE10 芎歸香蘇散 Cnidii, Angelicae Gigantis, Cyperi, and Perillae Powder	Decoction SY1 荊防敗毒散 Schizonepetae Spica and Saposhnikoviae Radix Toxin-Repelling Powder
After ulceration	TE19 淸肺瀉肝湯 Lung-Clearing Liver-Purging Decoction Exess heat: ◆ 承氣湯 Qi-Coordinating Decoction TE63 大黃散 Rhei Rhizoma Powder	SE15 十全大補湯 Ten Wholesome Greatly Tonifying Decoction SE6 補中益氣湯 Middle-Tonifying Qi-Replenishing Decoction SE74 人蔘散 Ginseng Radix Powder SE89 巴豆膏 Crotonis Semen Paste	SE5 黃連導白散 Coptidis Rhizoma White-Conducting Powder SY19 陽毒白虎湯 Yang Toxin White Tiger Decoction SY49 豚卵散 Pufferfish Roe Powder

47) Various Abscess

Symptom	Taeeum type	Soeum type	Soyang type
Inner abscess	TE1 太陰調胃湯 Taeeum Stomach-Regulating Decoction Excessive heat: ◆ 承氣湯 Qi-Coodrinating Decoction	SE4 人蔘官桂附子湯 Ginseng, Cinnamomi Cortex, and Aconiti Decoction SE15 十全大補湯 Ten Wholesome Greatly Tonifying Decoction	SY9 荊防地黃湯 Schizonepetae, Saposhnikoviae, and Rehmanniae Radix Preparata Decoction SY21 忍冬藤地骨皮湯 Lonicerae Caulis and Lycii Radicis Cortex Decoction

48) Gynecology and Obstetrics

Symptom	Taeeum type	Soeum type	Soyang type
Menstrual irregularities	Cold: TE1 太陰調胃湯 Taeeum Stomach-Regulating Decoction Heat: TE18 熱多寒少湯 Heat-Dominant Cold-Recessive Decoction	SE13 八物君子湯 Eight-Element Noble Decoction	SY43 生地黃湯 Rehmanniae Radix Crudus Decoction

Symptom	Taeeum type	Soeum type	Soyang type
Morning sickness	TE29 補肺元湯 Lung-Prime Tonifying Decoction TE7 經驗調胃湯 Empirical Stomach-Regulating Decoction	SE28 薑朮寬中湯 Zingiberis Rhizoma and Atractylodis Rhizoma Alba Middle-Soothing Decoction	SY4 荊防瀉白散 Schizonepetae Spica and Saposhnikoviae Radix White-Draining Powder
Vaginal bleeding during pregnancy	Cold: TE64 保胎飮 Fetus-Protecting Decoction Heat : TE65 文武保胎飮 Gentle-Firm Fetus-Protecting Decoction	SE90 加味八物湯 Eight-Element Added Decoction	SY62 保胎地黃湯 Fetus-Protecting Rehmanniae Radix Preparata Decoction
Threatened abortion	TE7 經驗調胃湯 Empirical Stomach-Regulating Decoction added Scutellaria Root 黃芩. TE57 千金文武湯 Thousand Gold Pieces Gentle-Firm Decoction TE29 補肺元湯 Lung-Prime Tonifying Decoction	SE6 補中益氣湯 Middle-Tonifying Qi-Replenishing Decoction ◆ 李氏補中益氣湯 Lee's Middle-Tonifying Qi-Replenishing Decoction	SY9 荊防地黃湯 Schizonepetae, Saposhnikoviae, and Rehmanniae Radix Preparata Decoction Fire: SY20 凉膈散火湯 Diaphragm-Cooling Fire-Dissipating Decoction
Early abortion	Cold: TE64 保胎飮 Fetus-Protecting Decoction Heat : TE65 文武保胎飮 Gentle-Firm Fetus-Protecting Decoction	SE90 加味八物湯 Eight-Element Added Decoction	SY62 保胎地黃湯 Fetus-Protecting Rehmanniae Radix Preparata Decoction
Promoting delivery	TE59 二門五味湯 Liriope, Asparagus, and Schisandrae Decoction	SE91 藿香正氣散 Agastachis Herba Qi-Correcting Powder Constitutional deficiency: SE13 八物君子湯 Eight-Element Noble Decoction	SY51 催生散 Delivery-Inducing Powder SY41 六味地黃湯 Six-Element Rehmanniae Radix Preparata Decoction
Retention of placenta	TE59 二門五味湯 Liriope, Asparagus, and Schisandrae Decoction	SE91 藿香正氣散 Agastachis Herba Qi-Correcting Powder	SY22 熟地黃苦蔘湯 Rehmanniae Radix Preparata and Sophorae Radix

Symptom	Taeeum type	Soeum type	Soyang type
	TE19 清肺瀉肝湯 Lung-Clearing Liver-Purging Decoction		Decoction
Expulsion of dead fetus	TE6 承氣調胃湯 Qi-Coordinating Stomach-Regulating Decoction	SE13 八物君子湯 Eight-Element Noble Decoction SE31 巴豆丹 Crotonis Semen Pellet	SY22 熟地黃苦蔘湯 Rehmanniae Radix Preparata and Sophorae Radix Decoction SY27 甘遂天一丸 Euphorbiae Kansui Radix Heaven-One Pill
Eclampsia of pregnancy	The prescription is the same as for the treatment of adults.		
Pregnancy vexation	The prescription is the same as for the pregnancy suspension section.	None	None
Pregnancy swelling, Strangury of pregnancy, Cough during pregnancy, Dysentery during pregnancy, Malaria during pregnancy	The prescription is the same as the treatment of adults.		
Pregnancy suspension	TE29 補肺元湯 Lung-Prime Tonifying Decoction	SE13 八物君子湯 Eight-Element Noble Decoction	SY41 六味地黃湯 Six-Element Rehmanniae Radix Preparata Decoction
Pregnancy aphasia, Cold damage	The prescription is the same as the treatment of adults.	The prescription is the same as the treatment of adults.	The prescription is the same as the treatment of adults.
Postpartum consumptive disease	TE1 太陰調胃湯 Taeeum Stomach-Regulating Decoction	SE13 八物君子湯 Eight-Element Noble Decoction SE15 十全大補湯 Ten Wholesome Greatly Tonifying Decoction	SY41 六味地黃湯 Six-Element Rehmanniae Radix Preparata Decoction
Postpartum abdominal pain	TE1 太陰調胃湯 Taeeum Stomach-Regulating Decoction	◆ 八物湯 Eight Ingredients Decoction added Angelicae Radix 當歸尾 and Cyperi Rhizoma	SY13 牧丹地黃湯 Moutan Cortex and Rehmanniae Radix Preparata Decoction added Sophorae Radix

Symptom	Taeeum type	Soeum type	Soyang type
	TE19 清肺瀉肝湯 Lung-Clearing Liver-Purging Decoction added Nelumbinis Semen 蓮肉 and Typhae Pollen 蒲黃	香附子	苦蔘 and Rehmanniae Radix Crudus 生地黃
Blood vertigo, flooding, epistaxis, cough, loss of voice, yin collapse, diarrhea, constipation, puffy swelling	The prescription is the same as with the treatment of adults.		
Feeling of oppression and dizziness	The prescription is the same as for the consumptive disease section.		
Hemorrhoids due to Wind	The prescription is the same as for the wind section.		

49) Pediatrics

Symptom	Taeeum type	Soeum type	Soyang type
Fright seizure	TE45 牛黃淸心元 Bovis Calculus Heart-Clearing Pill TE42 石菖蒲遠志散 Acori Graminei Rhizoma and Polygalae Radix Powder	SE55 蘇合香元 Styrax Liquides Pill SE28 薑朮寬中湯 Zingiberis Rhizoma and Atractylodis Rhizoma Alba Middle-Soothing Decoction	SY48 靈砂散 Vermilionum Powder SY26 朱砂益元散 Cinnabaris Prime-Replenishing Powder
Night crying	TE42 石菖蒲遠志散 Acori Graminei Rhizoma and Polygalae Radix Powder	SE55 蘇合香元 Styrax Liquides Pill SE28 薑朮寬中湯 Zingiberis Rhizoma and Atractylodis Rhizoma Alba Middle-Soothing Decoction	SY3 導赤降氣湯 Red-Conducting Qi-Lowering Decoction
Chronic infantile convulsion	TE29 補肺元湯 Lung-Prime Tonifying Decoction After occurring : The prescription is same	SE33 人蔘陳皮湯 Ginseng Radix and Citri Pericarpium Decoction SE34 人蔘桂皮湯	The prescription is same with the wind – emergency part.

Symptom	Taeeum type	Soeum type	Soyang type
	with the wind – emergency part.	Ginseng Radix and Cinnamomi Cortex Decoction	
Epilepsy	The prescription is same with the spirit part.		
Infantile malnutrition	TE18 熱多寒少湯 Heat-Dominant Cold-Recessive Decoction	SE13 八物君子湯 Eight-Element Noble Decoction	SY45 李氏肥兒丸 Lee's Child-Plumping Pill
Various types of fever, Vomitting and diarrhea, Common cold, Rapid dyspnea, Diarrhea and dysentery, Abdominal pain, Abdominal distention.	The prescription is the same as with the treatment of adults.		
Intestinal pain	TE42 石菖蒲遠志散 Acori Graminei Rhizoma and Polygalae Radix Powder	SE18 香附子八物湯 Cyperi Rhizoma Eight-Element Decoction	SY2 荊防導赤散 Schizonepetae Spica and Saposhnikoviae Radix Red-Conducting Powder
Pigeon chest	TE18 熱多寒少湯 Heat-Dominant Cold-Recessive Decoction	SE13 八物君子湯 Eight-Element Noble Decoction	SY1 荊防敗毒散 Schizonepetae Spica and Saposhnikoviae Radix Toxin-Repelling Powder
Tortoise back	TE1 太陰調胃湯 Taeeum Stomach-Regulating Decoction	SE91 藿香正氣散 Agastachis Herba Qi-Correcting Powder	SY1 荊防敗毒散 Schizonepetae Spica and Saposhnikoviae Radix Toxin-Repelling Powder
Ununited skull	TE10 腎氣調胃湯 Kidney Qi Stomach-Regulating Decoction	SE13 八物君子湯 Eight-Element Noble Decoction double added Atractylodis Rhizoma Alba 白朮	SY41 六味地黃湯 Six-Element Rehmanniae Radix Preparata Decoction SY1 荊防敗毒散 Schizonepetae Spica and Saposhnikoviae Radix Toxin-Repelling Powder
Protruding fontanel	TE1 太陰調胃湯 Taeeum Stomach-Regulating	SE10 芎歸香蘇散 Cnidii, Angelicae Gigantis, Cyperi, and	SY4 荊防瀉白散 Schizonepetae Spica and Saposhnikoviae

Symptom	Taeeum type	Soeum type	Soyang type
	Decoction	Perillae Powder SE13 八物君子湯 Eight-Element Noble Decoction	Radix White-Draining Powder
Sunken fontanel	TE1 太陰調胃湯 Taeeum Stomach-Regulating Decoction ◆ 葛茸大補湯 Puerariae Surculus Greatly Tonifying Decoction	SE6 補中益氣湯 Middle-Tonifying Qi-Replenishing Decoction SE15 十全大補湯 Ten Wholesome Greatly Tonifying Decoction SE5 升陽益氣湯 Yang-Upraising Qi-Replenishing Decoction	SY9 荊防地黃湯 Schizonepetae, Saposhnikoviae, and Rehmanniae Radix Preparata Decoction SY40 李氏凉膈散 Lee's Diaphragm-Cooling Powder SY45 李氏肥兒丸 Lee's Child-Plumping Pill
Five stiffnesses	Cold : TE9 調胃續命湯 Stomach-Regulating Life-Prolonging Decoction Heat : TE19 清肺瀉肝湯 Lung-Clearing Liver-Purging Decoction	SE9 川芎桂枝湯 Cnidii Rhizoma and Cinnamomi Ramulus Decoction SE18 香附子八物湯 Cyperi Rhizoma Eight-Element Decoction	SY1 荊防敗毒散 Schizonepetae Spica and Saposhnikoviae Radix Toxin-Repelling Powder SY20 凉膈散火湯 Diaphragm-Cooling Fire-Dissipating Decoction
Retardation in tooth growth	TE10 腎氣調胃湯 Kidney Qi Stomach-Regulating Decoction	SE15 十全大補湯 Ten Wholesome Greatly Tonifying Decoction	SY9 荊防地黃湯 Schizonepetae, Saposhnikoviae, and Rehmanniae Radix Preparata Decoction
Erysipelas	The prescription is the same as the skin section.		
Various types of sores	The prescription is the same as the Abscess and Carbuncle section.		
Smallpox and measles	Deficiency pattern should be treated with supplementation; excess pattern should be treated with drainage; cold pattern should be treated with warmth; and heat pattern should be treated with cold. Do not carelessly treat with Toxin-Resolving or Exterior-Resolving drugs. Otherwise, source qi must be damaged and the state becomes more unfavorable.		
Early fever (Protrusion with formation of pus)	It should be treated according to the treatment of cold-damage six-meridian disease.		
Scar formation	It should be treated according to the treatment of cold-damage six-meridian disease.		

<table>
<tr><th>Symptom</th><th>Taeeum type</th><th>Soeum type</th><th>Soyang type</th></tr>
<tr><td>Smallpox fright convulsion, Smallpox vomiting, Smallpox diarrhea, Smallpox vexing thirst, Smallpox shivering, Smallpox aphasia, Smallpox in pregnancy</td><td colspan="3">It should be treated according to the treatment of six meridian disease.</td></tr>
<tr><td>Measles</td><td colspan="3">It should be treated according to the treatment of six meridian disease.</td></tr>
<tr><td>Measles in pregnancy</td><td colspan="3">It should be treated according to the treatment of six meridian disease.</td></tr>
</table>

Sasang Formulas and Prescriptions
東醫四象新編劑方

Taeeum Type 太陰人

TE1 Taeeum Stomach-Regulating Decoction Taeeumjowi-tang 太陰調胃湯

Used to treat jaundice, cold damage, seasonal headache, generalized pain, absence of sweating, food stagnation, feeling of fullness, and weakness in the legs.

薏苡仁 Coicis Semen 11.25g
乾栗 Castaneae Semen 11.25g
萊菔子 Raphani Semen 7.5g
五味子 Schisandrae Fructus 3.75g
麥門冬 Liriopis Tuber 3.75g
石菖蒲 Acori Graminei Rhizoma 3.75g
桔梗 Platycodonis Radix 3.75g
麻黃 Ephedrae Herba 3.75g

To treat yin collapse, add 民魚膠, 脯 air bladder or jerky of Leiocassis Longirostris. It is called TE2 Hwaseokjowi-tang 花惜調胃湯 Piteous Flower Stomach-Regulating Decoction.
To treat cough, add 麻黃 Ephedrae Herba 11.75g. It is called TE3 Mahwangjowi-tang 麻黃調胃湯 Ephedrae Herba Stomach-Regulating Decoction.
To treat diarrhea, add 樗根皮 Ailanthi Cortex 7.5g. It is called TE4 Gogijowi-tang 固氣調胃湯 Qi-Securing Stomach-Regulating Decoction.
To treat absence of sweating, add 升麻 Cimicifugae Rhizoma and 白芷 Angelicae Dahuricae Radix. It is called TE5 Seungjijowi-tang 升芷調胃湯 Cimicifugae Rhizoma and Angelicae Dahuricae Radix Stomach-Regulating Decoction.
To treat blocked flow of feces and delirious speech due to dominant heat, remove 薏苡仁 Coicis Semen, 乾栗 Castaneae Semen, and add 乾葛 Puerariae Radix 18.75g, 大黃 Rhei Rhizoma 11.25g, 藁本 Angelicae Tenuissimae Radix 7.5g. It is called TE6 Seunggijowi-tang 承氣調胃湯 Qi-Coordinating Stomach-Regulating Decoction.
To treat lung and kidney deficiency in pregnant women, remove 薏苡仁 Coicis Semen, 萊菔子 Raphani Semen, and add Pini Koraiensis Semen 7.5g. It is called TE7 Gyeonghumjowi- tang 經驗調胃湯 Empirical Stomach-Regulating Decoction.
To treat absence of sweating, and cold-heat, add 升麻 Cimicifugae Rhizoma and 黃芩 Scutellariae Radix. It is called TE8 Seunggeumjowi-tang 升芩調胃湯 Cimicifugae Rhizoma and Scutellariae Radix Stomach-Regulating Decoction.
To treat wind syndrome, 藁本 Angelicae Tenuissimae Radix must to be changed into 五味子 Schisandrae Fructus. It is called TE9 Jowisongmyung-tang 調胃續命湯 Stomach-Regulating Life-Prolonging Decoction.
To treat kidney yang deficiency, add 海松子 Pini Koraiensis Semen 7.5g. It is called TE10 Singijowi-tang 腎氣調胃湯 Kidney Qi Stomach-Regulating Decoction.

TE11

Puerariae Radix Flesh-Resolving Decoction

Galgeunhaegi-tang 葛根解肌湯

Used to treat yang-toxin, reddened complexion like silken texture, sore throat, spitting out pus and blood.

- Also used to treat mild aversion to cold, fever, pain in the eyes, dry nose, sweating with tidal fever, blocked or astringed flow of feces, wasting-thirst, madness and delirium, abdominal pain, spontaneous diarrhea, continuous fever due to epidemic cold, pestilence, cold syncope continuing five days with absence of sweating.

葛根 Puerariae Radix 11.25g
升麻 Cimicifugae Rhizoma 7.5g
黃芩 Scutellariae Radix 5.625g
杏仁 Armeniacae Semen 5.625g
桔梗 Platycodonis Radix 3.75g
酸棗仁(炒) Zizyphi Semen (stir-bake) 3.75g
大黃 Rhei Rhizoma 3.75g
白芷 Angelicae Dahuricae Radix 3.75g

TE12

Stomach-Regulating Upraising-Clearing Decoction

Jowiseungcheong-tang 調胃升淸湯

Used to treat stuffiness and fullness after eating, weakness in legs, middle wasting-thirst, excessive appetite due to middle wasting-thirst.

薏苡仁 Coicis Semen 11.25g
乾栗 Castaneae Semen 11.25g
萊菔子 Raphani Semen 5.625g
麻黃 Ephedrae Herba 3.75g
桔梗 Platycodonis Radix 3.75g
麥門冬 Liriopis Tuber 3.75g
五味子 Schisandrae Fructus 3.75g
石菖蒲 Acori Graminei Rhizoma 3.75g
遠志 Polygalae Radix 3.75g
天門冬 Asparagi Tuber 3.75g
酸棗仁 Zizyphi Semen 3.75g
龍眼肉 Longan Arillus 3.75g

When 薏苡仁 Coicis Semen and 萊菔子 Raphani Semen are removed, and 海松子 Pini Koraiensis Semen are added, it is called TE13 Gyeongheomseungcheong-tang 經驗升淸湯 Empirical Upraising-Clearing Decoction.
When 海松子 Pini Koraiensis Semen is removed and 杏仁 Armeniacae Semen 3.75g added, it is called TE14 Haenginseungcheong-tang 杏仁升淸湯 Armeniacae Semen Upraising- Clearing Decoction.

TE15 Heart-Clearing Nelumbinis Semen Decoction
Cheongsimyeonja-tang 清心蓮子湯

Used to treat dream ejaculation due to consumptive disease, abdominal pain and diarrhea, curled tongue due to wind stroke, pain from chest to abdomen due to food stagnation.

蓮肉 Nelumbinis Semen 7.5g
山藥 Dioscoreae Rhizoma 7.5g
天門冬 Asparagi Tuber 7.5g
麥門冬 Liriopis Tuber 7.5g
遠志 Polygalae Radix 7.5g
石菖蒲 Acori Graminei Rhizoma 7.5g
山棗仁 Zizyphi Semen 7.5g
龍眼肉 Longan Arillus 7.5g
栢子仁 Thujae Semen 7.5g
黃芩 Scutellariae Radix 7.5g
萊菔子 Raphani Semen 7.5g
甘菊 Chrysanthemi Flos 1.125g

TE16 Ephedrae Herba Panting-Stabilizing Decoction
Mahwangjeongcheon-tang 麻黃定喘湯

Used to treat pain in the chest and abdomen, and panting.

麻黃 Ephedrae Herba 11.25g
杏仁 Armeniacae Semen 5.625g
黃芩 Scutellariae Radix 3.75g
萊菔子 Raphani Semen 3.75g
桑白皮 Mori Cortex 3.75g
桔梗 Platycodonis Radix 3.75g
麥門冬 Liriopis Tuber 3.75g
款冬花 Farfarae Flos 3.75g
白果(炒黃) Ginkgonis Semen (stir-bake to yellow) 20pcs

TE17 Ephedrae Herba Pain-Stabilizing Decoction
Mahwangjeongtong-tang 麻黃定痛湯

Used to treat pain in the chest and abdomen.

薏苡仁 Coicis Semen 11.25g
麻黃 Ephedrae Herba 7.5g
萊菔子 Raphani Semen 7.5g
杏仁 Armeniacae Semen 3.75g
石菖蒲 Acori Graminei Rhizoma 3.75g
桔梗 Platycodonis Radix 3.75g
麥門冬 Liriopis Tuber 3.75g
五味子 Schisandrae Fructus 3.75g
使君子 Quisqualis Fructus 3.75g
龍肉 Longan Arillus 3.75g
栢下仁 Thujae Semen 3.75g
乾栗 Castaneae Semen 7 kernels

TE18 Heat-Dominant Cold-Recessive Decoction Yeoldahanso-tang 熱多寒少湯

Used to treat dream ejaculation due to consumptive disease continued for three or four days.

葛根 Puerariae Radix 15g
黃芩 Scutellariae Radix 7.5g
藁本 Angelicae Tenuissimae Radix 7.5g
萊菔子 Raphani Semen 3.75g
桔梗 Platycodonis Radix 3.75g
升麻 Cimicifugae Rhizoma 3.75g
白芷 Angelicae Dahuricae Radix 3.75g

To treat constipation, add 3.75g of 大黃 Rhei Rhizoma. It is called TE19 Cheongpyesagan-tang 淸肺瀉肝湯 Lung-Clearing Liver-Purging Decoction.
If there is not constipation everyday, remove 大黃 Rhei Rhizoma and add 龍骨 Fossilia Ossis Mastodi. This prescription is called TE20 Jeongsinsagan-tang 定神瀉肝湯 Spirit-Stabilizing Liver-Purging Decoction.
To treat nausea and vomiting, vexation and heavy feeling of dizziness due to heat syndrome, red and yellow complexion, blackened hand-finger, puffy swelling in palm and dorsum of hand, and weakness of the limbs, add 大黃 Rhei Rhizoma.
To treat drinking water due to dryness and thirst, constipation, frequent urination as if to drink 10L of water and to make 10L of urination, add 藁本 Angelicae Tenuissimae Radix and 大黃 Rhei Rhizoma.
• It is also used to treat dry throat and diarrhea.

TE21 Cold-Dominant Heat-Recessive Decoction Handayeolso-tang 寒多熱少湯

Used to treat cold syncope continued four or five days and absence of sweating.

薏苡仁 Coicis Semen 11.25g
萊菔子 Raphani Semen 7.5g
麥門冬 Liriopis Tuber 3.75g
桔梗 Platycodonis Radix 3.75g
黃芩 Scutellariae Radix 3.75g
杏仁 Armeniacae Semen 3.75g
麻黃 Ephedrae Herba 3.75g
乾栗 Castaneae Semen 7 kernels

When five or seven pieces of 蠐螬 Holotrichia is added, it is called TE22 Jejopaedok- san 蠐螬敗毒散 Holotrichiae Vermis Toxin-Repelling Powder. It is used to treat efflux diarrhea.
To treat dry stool, remove 薏苡仁 Coicis Semen and 乾栗 Castaneae Semen, and add 葛根 Puerariae Radix and 大黃 Rhei Rhizoma. It is called TE23 Yunpyecheonggan-tang 潤肺淸肝湯 Lung-Moistening Liver-Clearing Decoction.

TE24 Galgeunseunggi-tang 葛根承氣湯

Puerariae Radix Qi-Coordinating Decoction

Used to treat loathing of cold and high fever due to warm disease, and dry stool.

- Painful redness of the head, face, neck and cheek.
- Loss of appetite, delirious speech, and mania due to interior heat. Reversal cold of the hands and in flexible legs after extending because heat creates wind.
- Blocked flow of feces.

葛根 Puerariae Radix 15g
大黃 Rhei Rhizoma 7.5g
黃芩 Scutellariae Radix 7.5g
桔梗 Platycodonis Radix 3.75g
升麻 Cimicifugae Rhizoma 3.75g
白芷 Angelicae Dahuricae Radix 3.75g

To treat retention of the placenta, add 7.5g of 黃芩 Scutellariae Radix to Gleditsiae Spina Decoction 皂角湯, It is called TE25 Galgeundaeseunggi-tang 葛根大承氣湯 Puerariae Radix Major Qi-Coordinating Decoction
When 7.5g of 萊菔子 Raphani Semen is added to TE25 Galgeundaeseunggi-tang 葛根大承氣湯 Puerariae Radix Major Qi-Coordinating Decoction, it is called TE26 Naebokjaseunggi-tang 萊菔子承氣湯 Raphani Semen Qi-Coordinating Decoction.

TE27 Joripyewon-tang 調理肺元湯

Lung-Prime Regulating Decoction

Used to regulate after releasing severe disease.

麥門冬 Liriopis Tuber 7.5g
桔梗 Platycodonis Radix 7.5g
薏苡仁 Coicis Semen 7.5g
黃芩 Scutellariae Radix 3.75g
麻黃 Ephedrae Herba 3.75g
萊菔子 Raphani Semen 3.75g

TE28 Mahwangbalpyo-tang 麻黃發表湯

Ephedrae Herba Exterior-Effusing Decoction

Used to treat greater yang pattern; absence of sweating and panting. Or add 3.75g of 升麻 Cimicifugae Rhizoma, 3 units of 白果 Ginkgonis Semen.

桔梗 Platycodonis Radix 11.25g
麻黃 Ephedrae Herba 5.625g
麥門冬 Liriopis Tuber 3.75g
黃芩 Scutellariae Radix 3.75g
杏仁 Armeniacae Semen 3.75g

TE29 Lung-Prime Tonifying Decoction
Bopyewon-tang 補肺元湯

Used to treat infantile diarrhea. If it occurs more than ten times, there must be chronic infantile convulsions. This disease pattern can be prevented with the prescription.

麥門冬 Liriopis Tuber 11.25g
桔梗 Platycodonis Radix 7.5g
五味子 Schisandrae Fructus 3.75g

To treat epistaxis, add 3.75g of 山藥 Dioscoreae Rhizoma, 3.75g of 薏苡仁 Coicis Semen, and 3.75g of 萊菔子 Raphani Semen. It is called TE30 Sanyakbopyewon- tang 山藥補肺元湯 Dioscoreae Rhizoma Lung-Prime Tonifying Decoction.

TE31 Polaris-Aspiring Black Vitality Pellet
Gongjinheugwon-dan 拱辰黑元丹

Used to treat the weak patient who has interior symptom and cold symptom.

鹿茸 Cervi Parvum Cornu 150g, 187.5g or 225g
山藥 Dioscoreae Rhizoma 150g
天門冬 Asparagi Tuber 150g
蠐螬 Holotrichia 37.5~75g
麝香 Moschus 18.75g

Boil the flesh of Mume Fructus and puree into a soft paste. Together with the other pulverized drugs, make the pills as big as the seed of an empress tree. Take 50~70 pills for each dose with warm water or liquor.

TE32 Cervi Parvum Cornu Greatly Tonifying Decoction
Nokyongdaebo-tang 鹿茸大補湯

Used to treat the weak patient displaying exterior patterns and cold patterns.

鹿茸 Cervi Parvum Cornu 7.5g, 11.25g, or 15g
麥門冬 Liriopis Tuber 5.625g
薏以仁 Coicis Semen 5.625g
山藥 Dioscoreae Rhizoma 3.75g
天門冬 Asparagi Tuber 3.75g
五味子 Schisandrae Fructus 3.75g
杏仁 Armeniacae Semen 3.75g
麻黃 Ephedrae Herba 3.75g

TE33

Gleditsiae Fructus and Rhei Rhizoma Decoction

Jogakdaehwang-tang 皀角大黃湯

Used to treat loathing of cold and high fever, dry stool, red swelling of the head, face, neck, and cheek.

升麻 Cimicifugae Rhizoma 11.25g
葛根 Puerariae Radix 11.25g
大黃 Rhei Rhizoma 3.75g
皀角 Gleditsiae Fructus 3.75g

Do not use this medicine over three or four packs. The potency of this drug is extremely strong.

TE34

Puerariae Radix and Spirodelae Herba Decoction

Galgeunbupyeong-tang 葛根浮萍湯

Used to treat puffy swelling due to interior heat.

葛根 Puerariae Radix 11.25g
萊菔子 Raphani Semen 7.5g
黃芩 Scutellariae Radix 7.5g
大黃 Rhei Rhizoma 3.75g
浮萍(紫背) Spirodelae Herba (with purple backs) 3.75g
蠐螬 Holotrichia 10 pcs

When 7.5g of Angelicae Tenuissimae Radix is added, it is called TE35 Gobonbupyeong-tang 藁本浮萍湯 Puerariae Radix and Spirodelae Herba Decoction.
When 7.5g of 鹿茸 Cervi Parvum Cornu is added and 蠐螬 Holotrichia Vermis is removed, it is called TE36 Galyongbupyeong-tang 葛茸浮萍湯 Puerariae, Cervi Parvum Cornu, and Spirodelae Decoction.

TE37

Castaneae Semen and Holotrichia Vermis Decoction

Geonyuljejo-tang 乾栗蠐螬湯

Used to treat puffy swelling and the exterior patterns with more chills than fever.

乾栗 Castaneae Semen 100 units
蠐螬 Holotrichia Vermis 100 units

Take these as a decoction or stir-bake them with an adjuvant.

TE38 Castaneae Semen and Ailanthi Cortex Decoction Geonyuljeogeunpi-tang 乾栗樗根皮湯

Used to treat dysentery.

乾栗 Castaneae Semen 37.5g 樗根皮 Ailanthi Cortex 11.25-18.75g

Take this as a decoction or pills.

TE39 Melonis Calyx Powder Gwache-san 苽蔕散

Used to treat sudden stroke with congested sounds emanating from the chest and blankly staring into space.

苽蔕 Melonis Pedicellus (stir-bake to yellow)

Pulverize the above drug into powder of 1.125 or 1.875g. Take it with warm water. Or decoct 3.75g of milk and use it as a substitute of warm water.

TE40 Fel Ursi Powder Wungdam-san 熊膽散

Used to treat cold syncope for six or seven days and absence of sweating due to sudden stroke, and spasm of the extremities.

熊膽 Fel Ursi 1.125-1.875g

This prescription should be taken with warm water.

TE41 Moschus Powder Sahyang-san 麝香散

Used to treat vomiting and diarrhea due to poisoning.
- Acute abdominal pain
- This prescription should be taken with warm water or warm liquor.

麝香 Moschus 1.125-1.875g

TE42 Acori Graminei Rhizoma and Polygalae Radix Powder Seokchangpowonji-san 石菖蒲遠志散

Used to treat clenched jaw due to sudden infantile convulsion.

- Closed eyes and spasm of the extremities.
- This prescription should be taken with warm water. Another way is to take the powder of 遠志 Polygalae Radix and 石菖蒲 Acori Graminei Rhizoma with warm water and breathe the powder of 猪牙皀角 Gleditsiae Spina into the nasal cavity.

遠志(末) Polygalae Radix (pulverized) 37.5g
石菖蒲(末) Acori Graminei Rhizoma (pulverized) 3.75g
猪牙皀角(末) Gleditsiae Spina (pulverized) 1.125g

When 皀角 Gleditsiae Spina is removed and 3.75g of 龍骨 Fossilia Ossis Mastodi are added, it is called TE43 Samsin-san 三神散 Three Spirit Powder. This prescription should be taken with warm water.

TE44 Liriopis Tuber and Polygalae Radix Powder Maekmundongwonji-san 麥門冬遠志散

Used to make ears and eyes sharp and bright.

麥門冬 Liriopis Tuber 11.25g
遠志 Polygalae Radix 3.75g
石菖蒲 Acori Graminei Rhizoma 3.75g
五味子 Schisandrae Fructus 1.875g

TE45 Bovis Calculus Heart-Clearing Pill Wuhwangcheongsim-hwan 牛黃淸心元

Used to treat sudden wind stroke with loss of consciousness, congestion of phlegm and drool, clouding and fretting of essence-spirit, sluggish speech, paralysis of the limbs, and closed eyes.

山藥 Dioscoreae Rhizoma 26.25g
犀角 Rhinoceri Cornu 7.5g
蒲黃(炒) Typhae Pollen (stir-bake) 13.125g
大豆黃卷(炒) Glycine Semen Germinatum (stir-bake) 6.375g
麥門冬(去心) Liriopis Tuber (core-removed) 5.625g
黃芩 Scutellariae Radix 5.625g
桔梗 Platycodonis Radix 5.625g
杏仁(去皮尖) Armeniacae Semen (tip of the cortex removed) 5.625g
牛黃 Bovis Calculus 4.5g
羚羊角 Antelopis Cornu 3.75g
龍腦 Borneolum 3.75g
麝香 Moschus 3.75g
白斂 Ampelopsis Radix 2.625g
金箔 Aurum Foil 70 foils (20 foils of Aurum Foil are used to wrap the pills)
烏梅 Mume Fructus 20 unit

Make a soft extract of twenty 烏梅 Mume Fructus, steamed and pared. Pound the above drugs into a powder, knead it with the soft extract of the 烏梅 Mume Fructus and, from 37.5g of the mixture, make twenty pills wrapped in thin sheets of gold. Take one pill for each dose with warm water.

TE46 Acori Graminei Rhizoma and Polygalae Radix Powder[8)] Seokchangpowonji-san 石菖蒲遠志散

Used to make ears and eyes sharp and bright.

石菖蒲 Acori Graminei Rhizoma equal amount
遠志 Polygalae Radix Powder equal amount

Pulverize the above drugs into powder. Take 3.75g of this prescription with liquor three times a day.

TE47 Black Ustilago Pill Heunno-hwan 黑奴丸

Used to treat patients with macula caused by yang type inflammatory swelling or with a case of deteriorated loss of consciousness. They can still be treated on the condition that there is warmth in the epigastric region. Administer the following medicine by mouth.

麻黃 Ephedrae Herba 75g
大黃 Rhei Rhizoma 75g
黃芩 Scutellariae Radix 37.5g
釜底煤 Cauldron soot 37.5g
芒硝 Natrii Sulfas 37.5g
煙突墨 Furnace ash 37.5g
梁上塵 Dust (on the girder) 37.5g
小麥奴 Smutted ear of barley 37.5g

Pound the above drugs into a powder and make pills the size of bullets, then take one pill with spring water. After a short bout of shivering and sweating, the patient will recover.

- When 芒硝 Natrii Sulfas is removed, it is called TE48 Leesiheunno-hwan 李氏黑奴丸 Lee's Black Ustilago Pill.

8) This prescription has different ingredients with TE42 *Seokchangpowonji-san* 石菖蒲遠志散.

TE49 Pulse-Activating Powder
Saengmaek-san 生脈散

If this prescription is drunk in summer instead of water boiled with burned rice, it will give energy.

麥門冬(去心) Liriopis Tuber (core-removed) 7.5g
五味子 Schisandrae Fructus 3.75g

TE50 Two Holy Suffering-Saving Pill
Iseonggugo-hwan 二聖救苦丸

Used to treat seasonal epidemic disease.

大黃 Rhei Rhizoma 150g
牙皂 Gleditsiae Fructus 75g

Pulverize the above drugs into powder. Make 50 or 70 pills with flour paste the size of mung beans.
• One intake causes sweating.

TE51 Sallowness-Repelling Decoction
Toehwang-eum 退黃飮

Used to treat jaundice

牛肉 Beef (Caro Bovis)

It doesn't stick at the regular quantity. Make thick soup or eat it raw.

TE52 Immediate Effect Powder
Iphyo-san 立效散

Used to treat eye disease.

升麻 Cimicifugae Rhizoma equal amount
葛根 Puerariae Radix equal amount
白芷 Angelicae Dahuricae Radix equal amount
石菖蒲 Acori Graminei Rhizoma equal amount

Decoct and wash a lesion with this.

TE53 Marvelous Incense Stick Yeosin-ju 如神炷

Used to treat pain in the wind-gum or caries of the teeth.
• Hemilateral and vertex headache.

大黃 Rhei Rhizoma 3.75g
藁本 Angelicae Tenuissimae Radix 3.75g
升麻 Cimicifugae Rhizoma 3.75g
皂角 Gleditsiae Fructus 3.75g
麻黃 Ephedrae Herba 3.75g

Pulverize the above drugs into powder and curl them with paper. Make seven sticks and fume into the nose. Then yellow water will pass from nose.

TE54 Kidney-Restoring Brightening Polish Guisinilchalgwang 歸腎一擦光

Used to treat toothache due to kidney deficiency.

海松子(去殼) Pini Semen(shell removed)

It doesn't stick at the regular quantity. Attach this medicine to a painful tooth or steam from lower side.

TE55 Phlegm-Sluicing Decoction Gondam-tang 滾痰湯

萊菔子 Raphani Semen 37.5g

Extract juice by crushing.

It doesn't stick at the regular quantity. Attach this medicine to a painful tooth or steam from lower side.

TE56 Wind-Dispelling Speech-Releasing Powder
Geopunghaeeo-san 祛風解語散

Used to treat wind stroke with loss of speech.

升麻 Cimicifugae Rhizoma equal amount
白芷 Angelicae Dahuricae Radix equal amount
麻黃 Ephedrae Herba equal amount
藁本 Angelicae Tenuissimae Radix equal amount
菊花 Chrysanthemi Flos equal amount

Decoct the medicines with water and put them under a table to fumigate for nose. The patient will be able to speak long time later.

TE57 Thousand Gold Pieces Gentle-Firm Decoction
Cheongeummunmu-tang 千金文武湯

Used to treat dryness-heat of pregnant women who urinate two as they drink one.

葛根 Puerariae Radix 7.5g
山藥 Dioscoreae Rhizoma 7.5g
黃芩 Scutellariae Radix 7.5g
藁本 Angelicae Tenuissimae Radix 7.5g
麥門冬 Liriopis Tuber 3.75g
五味子 Schisandrae Fructus 3.75g
桔梗 Platycodonis Radix 3.75g
升麻 Cimicifugae Rhizoma 3.75g
白芷 Angelicae Dahuricae Radix 3.75g

TE58 Ten Thousand Gold Pieces Gentle-Firm Decoction
Mangeummunmu-tang 萬金文武湯

Used to treat lung wasting-thirst.

葛根 Puerariae Radix 15g
海松子 Pini Semen 40 pcs
黃芩 Scutellariae Radix 7.5g
藁本 Angelicae Tenuissimae Radix 7.5g
天門冬 Asparagi Tuber 3.75g
麥門冬 Liriopis Tuber 3.75g
五味子 Schisandrae Fructus 3.75g
桔梗 Platycodonis Radix 3.75g
升麻 Cimicifugae Rhizoma 3.75g
白芷 Angelicae Dahuricae Radix 3.75g
大黃 Rhei Rhizoma 3.75g
萊菔子 Raphani Semen 3.75g

TE59 Liriope, Asparagus, and Schisandrae Decoction
Imunomi-tang 二門五味湯

Used to treat difficult delivery or fecal block.

- When 葛根 Puerariae Radix, 大黃 Rhei Rhizoma, 萊菔子 Raphani Semen, and 升麻 Cimicifugae Rhizoma are added, this prescription can generally treat fecal and urinary block.

麥門冬 Liriopis Tuber 11.25g
天門冬 Asparagi Tuber 7.5g
五味子 Schisandrae Fructus 3.75g

TE60 Eye-Brightening Powder
Myeongmok-san 明目散

硼砂(製) Borax (processed)

Grind to a fine powder. Mix this prescription with milk, and drop to eyes.

TE61 Lung-Tonifying Lactation-Inducing Powder
Bopyetongyu-san 補肺通乳散

牛乳 Bovis Lac (Cow's milk) 1 unit
桔梗 Platycodonis Radix 37.5g
麻黃 Ephedrae Herba 37.5g
升麻 Cimicifugae Rhizoma 15g

牛乳 Bovis Lac can be changed with Cow's scrotum or four legs.

- Decoct 牛乳 Bovis Lac first, then put the three medicines into it and decoct together again. Administer randomly.

TE62 Three yellows Powder Samhwang-san 三黃散

Used to treat wrenched lumbar pain.

麻黃 Ephedrae Herba equal amount
黃芩 Scutellariae Radix equal amount
蒲黃 Typhae Pollen equal amount
石菖蒲 Acori Graminei Rhizoma equal amount
杏仁 Armeniacae Seme equal amount

Pulverize the above drugs. Take 7.5g of this prescription with warm liquor at a time.

TE63 Rhei Rhizoma Powder Daehwang-san 大黃散

Used to treat general sore.

大黃 Rhei Rhizoma equal amount
黃芩 Scutellariae Radix equal amount
杏仁 Armeniacae Semen equal amount
升麻 Cimicifugae Rhizoma equal amount
皀角 Gleditsiae Fructus equal amount
白斂 Ampelopsis Radix equal amount
白芷 Angelicae Dahuricae Radix equal amount

Pulverize the above drugs. This prescription should be taken with liquor.

TE64 Fetus-Protecting Decoction Botae-eum 保胎飮

Used to treat fetal bleeding due to cold.

乾栗 Castaneae Semen 11.25g
海松子 Pini Semen 7.5g
五味子 Schisandrae Fructus
麥門冬 Liriopis Tuber 5.625g
石菖蒲 Acori Graminei Rhizoma 5.625g
桔梗 Platycodonis Radix 5.625g
麻黃 Ephedrae Herba 5.625g
阿膠 Asini Corii Colla 5.625g
鹿角膠 Cervi Cornus Colla 5.625g
酸棗仁 Zizyphi Semen 3.75g
升麻 Cimicifugae Rhizoma 3.75g

TE65 Gentle-Firm Fetus-Protecting Decoction
Munmubotae-eum 文武保胎飮

Used to treat fetal bleeding due to more heat than cold.

葛根 Puerariae Radix 15g
山藥 Dioscoreae Rhizoma 7.5g
黃芩 Scutellariae Radix 7.5g
藁本 Angelicae Tenuissimae Radix 7.5g
麥門冬 Liriopis Tube 5.625g
天門冬 Asparagi Tuber 5.625g
五味子 Schisandrae Fructus 5.625g
桔梗 Platycodonis Radix 5.625g
升麻 Cimicifugae Rhizoma 5.625g
白芷 Angelicae Dahuricae Radix 5.625g
阿膠 Asini Corii Colla 5.625g
酸棗仁 Zizyphi Semen 5.625g
鹿角膠 Cervi Cornus Colla 5.625g

TE66 Lee's Qi-Coordinating Decoction
Leesiseunggi-tang 李氏承氣湯

Used to treat chest bind syndrome.

大黃 Rhei Rhizoma 15g
黃芩 Scutellariae Radix 7.5g
桔梗 Platycodonis Radix 3.75g
升麻 Cimicifugae Rhizoma 3.75g
白芷 Angelicae Dahuricae Radix 3.75g

Pulverize the above drugs. This prescription should be taken with liquor.

Empirical Prescriptions for Taeeum Type 太陰人 經驗方

TE-e1 Ephedrae Herba Metal-Water Decoction
Mahwanggeumsu-tang 麻黃金水湯

Used to treat headache and hasty panting due to cold damage.

麻黃 Ephedrae Herba 11.25g
欵冬花 Farfarae Flos 7.5g
麥門冬 Liriopis Tuber 7.5g
杏仁 Armeniacae Semen 3.75g
升麻 Cimicifugae Rhizoma 3.75g
桔梗 Platycodonis Radix 3.75g
葛根 Puerariae Radix 3.75g
黃芩 Scutellariae Radix 3.75g
五味子 Schisandrae Fructus 3.75g
白果 Ginkgonis Semen 10pcs.

TE-e2 Flesh-Resolving Greatly Relieving Decoction
Haegidaean-tang 解肌大安湯

Used to treat puffy swelling.

葛根 Puerariae Radix 15g
黃芩 Scutellariae Radix 3.75g
萊菔子 Raphani Semen 3.75g
藁本 Angelicae Tenuissimae Radix 3.75g
桔梗 Platycodonis Radix 3.75g
升麻 Cimicifugae Rhizoma 3.75g
白芷 Angelicae Dahuricae Radix 3.75g
蠐螬 Holotrichia 10pcs.

TE-e3 Cimicifugae Rhizoma Brain-Clearing Decoction
Seungmagaenoe-tang 升麻開腦湯

Used to treat cold reversal for 4 or 5 days, absence of sweating.

升麻 Cimicifugae Rhizoma 11.25g
麥門冬 Liriopis Tuber 3.75g
天門冬 Asparagi Tuber 3.75g
五味子 Schisandrae Fructus 3.75g
酸棗仁 Zizyphi Semen 3.75g
桔梗 Platycodonis Radix 3.75g
黃芩 Scutellariae Radix 3.75g
麻黃 Ephedrae Herba 3.75g
杏仁 Armeniacae Semen 3.75g
葛根 Puerariae Radix 3.75g
欵冬花 Farfarae Flos 3.75g
白芷 Angelicae Dahuricae Radix 3.75g
大黃 Rhei Rhizoma 3.75g

TE-e4

Asparagi Tuber Lung-Moistening Decoction

Cheonmundongyunpye-tang 天門冬潤肺湯

Used to treat eye pain, dry nose, increased cold and vigorous heat, headache, lumbago, and dryness and roughness.

天門冬 Asparagi Tuber 11.25g
黃芩 Scutellariae Radix 7.5g
麥門冬 Liriopis Tuber 3.75g
酸棗仁 Zizyphi Semen 3.75g
升麻 Cimicifugae Rhizoma 3.75g
葛根 Puerariae Radix 3.75g
桔梗 Platycodonis Radix 3.75g
五味子 Schisandrae Fructus 3.75g
大黃 Rhei Rhizoma 3.75g

TE-e5

Cervi Parvum Cornu Greatly Building Decoction

Nokyongdaejo-tang 鹿茸大造湯

Used to treat qi deficiency and tonify origin.

鹿茸 Cervi Parvum Cornu 7.5g
天門冬 Asparagi Tuber 7.5g
麥門冬 Liriopis Tuber 7.5g
升麻 Cimicifugae Rhizoma 3.75g
葛根 Puerariae Radix 3.75g
杏仁 Armeniacae Semen 3.75g
山棗仁 Zizyphi Semen 3.75g
黃芩 Scutellariae Radix 3.75g
五味子 Schisandrae Fructus 3.75g

TE-e6

Platycodonis Radix Pulse-Activating Powder

Gilgyeongsaengmaek-san 桔梗生脈散

Used to treat cold reversal for 4-5 days, absence of sweating, interior and exterior diseases.

麥門冬 Liriopis Tuber 11.25g
山藥 Dioscoreae Rhizoma 3.75g
桔梗 Platycodonis Radix 3.75g
黃芩 Scutellariae Radix 3.75g
黃栗 Dried Castaneae Semen 3.75g
五味子 Schisandrae Fructus 3.75g
白果 Ginkgonis Semen 3 pcs.

TE-e7

Heart-Clearing Dioscoreae Rhizoma Decoction

Cheongsimsanyak-tang 淸心山藥湯

Used to treat dream ejaculation due to consumptive disease, no abdominal pain, diarrhea, curled tongue impeding speech, and wind stroke.

山藥 Dioscoreae Rhizoma 11.25g
遠志 Polygalae Radix 7.5g
天門冬 Asparagi Tuber 3.75g
麥門冬 Liriopis Tuber 3.75g
蓮子肉 Nelumbinis Semen 3.75g
栢子仁 Thujae Semen 3.75g
酸棗仁 Zizyphi Semen 3.75g
龍肉 Longan Arillus 3.75g
桔梗 Platycodonis Radi 3.75g
黃芩 Scutellariae Radix 3.75g
石菖蒲 Acori Graminei Rhizoma 3.75g
菊花 Chrysanthemi Flos 1.875g

TE-e8

Gleditsiae Fructus Three Yellow Decoction

Jogaksamhwang-tang 皂角三黃湯

Used to treat slight cold and fever, eye pain, dry nose, vexation and thirst, delirious speech, red face due to yang toxin, red eye and sore throat, and spitting of blood.

大黃 Rhei Rhizoma 15g
黃芩 Scutellariae Radix 3.75g
麻黃 Ephedrae Herba 3.75g
升麻 Cimicifugae Rhizoma 3.75g
桔梗 Platycodonis Radix 3.75g
牙皂 Gleditsiae Fructus 3.75g

TE-e9

Spirodelae Herba and Rhei Rhizoma Decoction

Bupyeongdaehwang-tang 浮萍大黃湯

Used to treat cold damage exterior and interior pattern, acute constipation.

大黃 Rhei Rhizoma 15g
黃芩 Scutellariae Radix 7.5g
浮萍(紫背) Spirodelae Herba (with purple backs) 7.5g

TE-e10

Platycodonis Radix and Ailanthi Cortex Decoction

Gilgyeongjeogeunpi-tang 桔梗樗根皮湯

Used to treat dysentery with pus and blood.

樗根皮 Ailanthi Cortex 18.75g
桔梗 Platycodonis Radix 7.5g

Pulverize the above drugs. Make pills and take.

TE-e11 Dried Castaneae Semen Qi-Securing Decoction
Hwangyulgogi-tang 黃栗固氣湯

Used to treat glomus and fullness due to food stagnation, and weak legs.

黃栗 Castaneae Semen 100 units
桔梗 Platycodonis Radix 11.25g
五味子 Schisandrae Fructus 3.75g
樗根皮 Ailanthi Cortex 3.75g

TE-e12 Dried Castaneae Semen and Schisandrae Fructus Paste
Hwangyulomija-go 黃栗五味子膏

Used to treat abdominal distention and puffy swelling.
• Double the amount of prescription at the second time. And double the second one at the third time.

黃栗 Dried Castaneae Semen 100 units
五味子 Schisandrae Fructus 30 units

TE-e13 Bovis Calculus and Dioscoreae Rhizoma Pill
Wuhwangsanyak-won 牛黃山藥元

Used to treat wind stroke with loss of speech.

山藥 Dioscoreae Rhizoma 7.5g
遠志 Polygalae Radix 7.5g
牛黃 Bovis Calculus 0.75g

Make four pills and take with warm water.

TE-e14 Liriopis Tuber Decoction
Maekmundong-tang 麥門冬湯

Used to treat half-exterior and half interior patterns due to cold damage, exterior heat and diarrhea.

麥門冬 Liriopis Tuber 11.25g
葛根 Puerariae Radix 7.5g
桔梗 Platycodonis Radix 7.5g
薏苡仁 Coicis Semen 7.5g
黃芩 Scutellariae Radix 3.75g
萊菔子 Raphani Semen 3.75g
五味子 Schisandrae Fructus 3.75g

TE-e15 Armeniacae Semen and Liriopis Tuber Decoction
Haenginmaekmundong-tang 杏仁麥門冬湯

Used to treat eye disease and deafness.

杏仁 Armeniacae Semen 11.25g
麥門冬 Liriopis Tuber 11.25g
麻黃 Ephedrae Herba 3.75g
桔梗 Platycodonis Radix 3.75g
龍肉 Longan Arillus 3.75g
遠志 Polygalae Radix 3.75g
石菖蒲 Acori Graminei Rhizoma 3.75g
天門冬 Asparagi Tuber 3.75g
黃芩 Scutellariae Radix 3.75g
萊菔子 Raphani Semen 3.75g
五味子 Schisandrae Fructus 3.75g

TE-e16 Four Seasons Pellet
Sasi-dan 四時丹

Used to treat seasonal pestilence in yin and yang, exterior and interior, cold and heat, deficiency and excess patterns, food stagnation, pain from chest to abdomen, lung atrophy, strangury and malaria, jaundice, infantile malnutrition, red and white turbidity, and dream emission.

- And also used to treat aggregation-accumulation, fright epilepsy, vomiting and diarrhea, and cholera.
- This prescription is contraindicated for pregnant women.

大黃 Rhei Rhizoma 120g
皀角(炙) Gleditsiae Fructus (stir-bake with adjuvant) 15g
萊菔子 Raphani Semen 15g
杏仁 Armeniacae Semen 15g
石菖蒲 Acori Graminei Rhizoma 15g
使君子 Quisqualis Fructus 15g
五味子 Schisandrae Fructus 15g
犀角 Rhinoceri Cornu 15g
欵冬花 Farfarae Flos 15g
白歛 Ampelopsis Radix 15g
白芷 Angelicae Dahuricae Radix 15g
天門冬 Asparagi Tuber 15g
麥門冬 Liriopis Tuber 15g
桔梗 Platycodonis Radix 15g
麻黃 Ephedrae Herba 15g
升麻 Cimicifugae Rhizoma 15g
黃芩 Scutellariae Radix 15g
藁本 Ligustici Rhizoma 15g
蒲黃 Typhae Pollen 15g
黃栗 Dried Castaneae Semen 15g
浮萍 Spirodelae Herba 15g
蠐螬 Holotrichia 15g
龍腦 Borneolum Syntheticum 15g
山藥 Dioscoreae Rhizoma 15g

Pulverize the above drugs and make pills with decocted pulp of 烏梅 Mume Fructus. Make ten pills per 37.5g of this prescription. Take 36 pills with warm water.

TE-e17 Coicis Semen Stomach-Regulating Decoction Uiiinjowi-tang 薏苡仁調胃湯

Used to treat great and intemperate diarrhea.

薏苡仁 Coicis Semen 37.5g
乾栗 Castaneae Semen 7.5g
萊菔子 Raphani Semen 7.5g
麥門冬 Liriopis Tuber 3.75g
五味子 Schisandrae Fructus 3.75g
石菖蒲 Acori Graminei Rhizoma 3.75g
桔梗 Platycodonis Radix 3.75g
麻黃 Ephedrae Herba 3.75g

TE-e18 Rhei Rhizoma and Ailanthi Cortex Decoction Daehwangjeogeunpi-tang 大黃樗根皮湯

Used to dysentery.

大黃 Rhei Rhizoma 37.5 or 75g
樗根皮 Ailanthi Cortex 26.25g

TE-e19 Heart-Clearing Added Decoction Gamicheongsim-tang 加味淸心湯

Used to treat epistaxis, hematemesis, descent of blood, fearful throbbing.

• To treat generalized pain and vaginal discharge during menstrual periods, add 7.5g of 大黃 Rhei Rhizoma.

薏苡仁 Coicis Semen 18.75g
蓮肉 Nelumbinis Semen 7.5g
山藥 Dioscoreae Rhizoma 7.5g
天門冬 Asparagi Tuber 3.75g
麥門冬 Liriopis Tuber 3.75g
遠志 Polygalae Radix 3.75g
石菖蒲 Acori Graminei Rhizoma 3.75g
酸棗仁 Zizyphi Semen 3.75g
龍肉 Longan Arillus 3.75g
栢子仁 Thujae Semen 3.75g
黃芩 Scutellariae Radix 3.75g
萊菔子 Raphani Semen 3.75g
甘菊 Chrysanthemi Flos 1.125g

TE-e20 Cold-Recessive Added Decoction[9] Gamihanso-tang 加味寒少陽

Used to treat blood stasis pattern.

續斷 Dipsaci Radix 37.5g
葛根 Puerariae Radix 15g
黃芩 Scutellariae Radix 7.5g
藁本 Angelicae Tenuissimae Radix 7.5g
萊菔子 Raphani Semen 3.75g
桔梗 Platycodonis Radix 3.75g
升麻 Cimicifugae Rhizoma 3.75g
白芷 Angelicae Dahuricae Radix 3.75g

TE-e21 Platycodonis Radix Gilgyeong-tang 桔梗湯

Used to treat throat disease.

桔梗 Platycodonis Radix 11.25g
黃芩 Scutellariae Radix 7.5g
升麻 Cimicifugae Rhizoma 7.5g
白芷 Angelicae Dahuricae Radix 7.5g
麻黃 Ephedrae Herba 7.5g
藁本 Angelicae Tenuissimae Radix 7.5g
竹茹 Bambusae Caulis In Taeniam 7.5g

TE-e22 Heart-Clearing Added Decoction Gagamcheongsim-tang 加減清心湯

Used to treat stagnation and disturbing influence.

薏苡仁 Coicis Semen 11.25g
麻黃 Ephedrae Herba 11.25g
萊菔子 Raphani Semen 7.5g
蓮肉 Nelumbinis Semen 7.5g
桔梗 Platycodonis Radix 3.75g
麥門冬 Liriopis Tuber 3.75g
五味子 Schisandrae Fructus 3.75g
黃芩 Scutellariae Radix 3.75g
石菖蒲 Acori Graminei Rhizoma 3.75g

9) This is the prescription which 37.5g of 續斷 Dipsaci Radix is added to TE18 熱多寒少湯 Heat-Dominant Cold-Recessive Decoction.

TE-e23

Three Yellow Acori Graminei Rhizoma and Armeniacae Semen Powder

Samhwangseokin-san 三黃石仁散

Used to treat blood stasis lumbar pain.

麻黃 Ephedrae Herba 11.25g
大黃 Rhei Rhizoma 7.5g
黃芩 Scutellariae Radix 7.5g
石菖蒲 Acori Graminei Rhizoma 7.5g
杏仁 Armeniacae Semen 7.5g
皂角刺 Gleditsiae Spina 3.75g

TE-e24

Ascaris-Quieting Decoction

Anhoe-san 安蛔飮

Used to treat ascariasis.

乾栗 Castaneae Semen 26.25g
薏苡仁 Coicis Semen 26.25g
使君子 Quisqualis Fructus 5.625g
萊菔子 Raphani Semen 3.75g
石菖蒲 Acori Graminei Rhizoma 3.75g
白礬(半生半熟) Alumen (half-raw and half-boiled) 3.75g

TE-e25

Stomach-Regulating Added Decoction

Gamijowi-tang 加味調胃湯

Used to treat stagnation and disturbing influence.

海松子 Pini Koraiensis Semen 75g
升麻 Cimicifugae Rhizom 26.25g
薏苡仁 Coicis Semen 18.75g
麥門冬 Liriopis Tuber 7.5g
五味子 Schisandrae Fructus 3.75g
石菖蒲 Acori Graminei Rhizoma 3.75g
桔梗 Platycodonis Radix 3.75g
麻黃 Ephedrae Herba 3.75g

TE-e26 Platycodonis Radix Decoction (2) Gilgyeong-tang 桔梗湯

Used to treat block and repulsion.

桔梗 Platycodonis Radix 18.75g
杏仁 Armeniacae Semen 11.25g
麻黃 Ephedrae Herba 7.5g

TE-e27 Mume Fructus Decoction Omae-jeon 烏梅煎

Used to treat cough.

烏梅肉 Pulp of Mume Fructus 11.25g
桔梗 Platycodonis Radix 7.5g
杏仁 Armeniacae Semen 7.5g
桑白皮 Mori Cortex 5.625g
欵冬花 Farfarae Flos 5.625g
白果(炒) Ginkgonis Semen (stir-bake) 20 pcs.

TE-e28 Longan Arillus Stomach-Regulating Decoction Yongyukjowi-tang 龍肉調胃湯

Used to regulate the patient after major illness.

龍肉 Longan Arillus 37.5g
乾栗 Castaneae Semen 18.75g
栢子仁 Thujae Semen 7.5g
麥門冬 Liriopis Tuber 7.5g

TE-e29 Thousand Gold Pieces Stomach-Regulating Decoction Cheongeumjowi-tang 千金調胃湯

Used to treat epilepsy.

薏苡仁 Coicis Semen 26.25g
乾栗 Castaneae Semen 11.25g
遠志 Polygalae Radix 11.25g
石菖蒲 Acori Graminei Rhizoma 11.25g
麥門冬 Liriopis Tuber 7.5g
五味子 Schisandrae Fructus 7.5g
天門冬 Asparagi Tuber 7.5g
唐皀角 Gleditisiae Fructus 3.75g
桔梗 Platycodonis Radix 3.75g
麻黃 Ephedrae Herba 3.75g
蓮肉 Nelumbinis Semen 3.75g

Soeum Type 少陰人

SE1 Astragali, Cinnamomi Ramulus, and Aconiti Decoction
Hwanggigeyjibuja-tang 黃芪桂枝附子湯

Used to treat yang collapse.

黃芪 Astragali Radix 11.25g
桂枝 Cinnamomi Ramulus 11.25g
白芍藥 Paeoniae Radix Alba 7.5g
當歸 Angelicae Gigantis Radix 3.75 or 7.5g
大棗 Zizyphi Fructus 2 pulps
甘草(炙) Glycyrrhizae Radix et Rhizoma (stir-bake with honey) 3.75 or 7.5g
附子(炮) Aconiti Lateralis Radix Preparata 3.75 or 7.5g
生薑 Zingiberis Rhizoma Crudus 3 slices

SE2 Ginseng, Cinnamomi Ramulus, and Aconiti Decoction
Insamgeyjibuja-tang 人蔘桂枝附子湯

Also used to treat yang collapse.

人蔘 Ginseng Radix 15g
桂枝 Cinnamomi Ramulus 11.25g
白芍藥 Paeoniae Radix Alba 7.5g
黃芪 Astragali Radix 7.5g
當歸 Angelicae Gigantis Radix 3.75g
大棗 Zizyphi Fructus 2 pulps
甘草(炙) Glycyrrhizae Radix et Rhizoma (stir-bake with honey) 3.75g
附子(炮) Aconiti Lateralis Radix Preparata 3.75 or 7.5g
生薑 Zingiberis Rhizoma Crudus 3 slices

SE3 Yang-Upraising Qi-Replenishing Aconiti Lateralis Radix Preparata Decoction
Seungyangikgibuja-tang 升陽益氣附子湯

Also used to treat yang collapse.

人蔘 Ginseng Radix 7.5g
桂枝 Cinnamomi Ramulus 7.5g
白芍藥 Paeoniae Radix Alba 7.5g
黃芪 Astragali Radix 7.5g
白何烏 Polygoni Multiflori Radix Alba 3.75g
官桂 Cinnamomi Cortex 3.75g
當歸 Angelicae Gigantis Radix 3.75g
甘草 Glycyrrhizae Radix et Rhizoma 3.75g
附子 Aconiti Lateralis Radix Preparata 3.75g

SE4 Ginseng, Cinnamomi Cortex, and Aconiti Decoction
Insamgwangyebuja-tang 人蔘官桂附子湯

Used to treat yang collapse.

人蔘 Ginseng Radix 18.75g or 37.5g
官桂 Cinnamomi Cortex 11.25g
黃芪 Astragali Radix 11.25g
白芍藥 Paeoniae Radix Alba 7.5g
當歸 Angelicae Gigantis Radix 3.75g
甘草 Glycyrrhizae Radix et Rhizoma 3.75g
附子 Aconiti Lateralis Radix Preparata 3.75g or 7.5g

- The above four prescriptions (SE1, SE2, SE3, and SE4) are used for yang collapse, which is a critical disease. If the yang collapse patient's urine is clean and fluent, there is a possibility of recovery. The patient should take 3.75g of Aconiti Lateralis Radix Preparata twice a day. If he is in critical condition, with reddish and difficult urination, then there is little chance for recovery. The patient should take 7.5g of Aconiti Lateralis Radix Preparata two, three or four times a day. However, in general, before facing the critical condition, 3.75g of Aconiti Lateralis Radix Preparata should be taken. The same amount can also be used when the patient is recovering.
- If the patient has constipation, a kernel of 巴豆 Crotonis Semen should be used first, after that, the above four prescriptions should be used. It is a barometer that the patient has good bowel movements and lots of urine.

SE5 Yang-Upraising Qi-Replenishing Decoction
Seungyangikgi-tang 升陽益氣湯

Used to treat greater yang syndrome and early yang collapse syndrome; excessiveness in the stomach-intestines and late mania syndrome.

人蔘 Ginseng Radix 7.5g
桂枝 Cinnamomi Rhizoma 7.5g
黃芪 Astragali Radix 7.5g
白芍藥 Paeoniae Radix Alba 7.5g
官桂 Cinnamomi Cortex 3.75g
白何烏 Polygoni Multiflori Radix Alba 3.75g
當歸 Angelicae Gigantis Radix 3.75g
甘草(炙) Glycyrrhizae Radix et Rhizoma (stir-bake) 3.75g

SE6 Bojungikgi-tang 補中益氣湯

Middle-Tonifying Qi-Replenishing Decoction

Used to treat early pattern of yang collapse of greater yang syndrome; weekness due to overexertion and fatigue, heart vexation due to fever, spontaneous sweating, lower abdominal colic.

人蔘 Ginseng Radix 11.25g
黃芪 Astragali Radix 11.25g
白朮 Atractylodis Rhizoma Alba 3.75g
當歸 Angelicae Gigantis Radix 3.75g
陳皮 Citri Unshius Pericarpium 3.75g
甘草(炙) Glycyrrhizae Radix et Rhizoma (stir-bake) 3.75g
蘇葉 Perillae Folium 1.875g
藿香 Agastachis Herba 1.875g

To treat red nose syndrome, add 18.75g of 民魚脯 jerky of Leiocassis Longirostris and change 香附子 Cyperi Rhizoma into 當歸 Angelicae Gigantis Radix. It is called SE7 Gumihwasoek-tang 九味花惜湯 Nine-Flavor Piteous Flower Decoction.

SE8 Hwanggigyeji-tang 黃芪桂枝湯

Astragali Radix and Cinnamomi Ramulus Decoction

Used to treat yang collapse syndrome and early Ulgwang syndrome (Congestive-Hyperpsychotic syndrome).

桂枝 Cinnamomi Ramulus 11.25g
白芍藥 Paeoniae Radix Alba 7.5g
黃芪 Astragali Radix 7.5g
何烏 Polygoni Multiflori Radix Alba 3.75g
當歸 Angelicae Gigantis Radix 3.75g
甘草(炙) Glycyrrhizae Radix et Rhizoma (stir-bake) 3.75g
生薑 Zingiberis Rhizoma Crudus 3 slices
大棗 Zizyphi Fructus 2 pulps

SE9 Cheongunggyeji-tang 川芎桂枝湯

Cnidii Rhizoma and Cinnamomi Ramulus Decoction

Used to treat greater yang syndrome and early Ulgwang syndrome (Congestive-Hyperpsychotic syndrome).

桂枝 Cinnamomi Ramulus 11.25g
白芍藥 Paeoniae Radix Alba 11.25g
川芎 Cnidii Rhizoma 3.75g
蒼朮 Atractylodis Rhizoma 3.75g
陳皮 Citri Unshius Pericarpium 3.75g
甘草 Glycyrrhizae Radix et Rhizoma 3.75g

- Decoct the above drugs together and take them when there are malaria and aversion to cold.
- The patient with Ulgwang syndrome (Congestive-Hyperpsychotic syndrome) must be promoted sweating. Adding 3.75g of 蘇葉 Perillae Folium is better for promoting sweating.

SE10 Cnidii, Angelicae Gigantis, Cyperi, and Perillae Powder Gungguihyangso-san 芎歸香蘇散

Used to treat four seasons pestilence, greater yang syndrome, and yin desertion.

香附子 Cyperi Rhizoma 7.5g
紫蘇葉 Perillae Folium 3.75g
川芎 Cnidii Rhizoma 3.75g
當歸 Angelicae Gigantis Radix 3.75g
蒼朮 Atractylodis Rhizoma 3.75g
陳皮 Citri Unshius Pericarpium 3.75g
甘草 Glycyrrhizae Radix et Rhizoma 3.75g
生薑 Zingiberis Rhizoma Crudus 3 slices
大棗 Zizyphi Fructus 2 pulps
葱 Allii Fistulosi Bulbus 5 roots

When 18.75g of 民魚脯 jerky of Leiocassis Longirostris is added, it is called SE11 Bijeonhyangso-san 秘傳香蘇散 Secret Cyperi Rhizoma and Perillae Folium Powder.

SE12 Arisaematis Rhizoma and Aucklandiae Radix Qi-Correcting Powder[10] Seonghyangjeonggi-san 星香正氣散

Used to treat general wind stroke, qi stroke, phlegm syncope, crapulent syncope.

SE13 Eight-Element Noble Decoction Palmulgunja-tang 八物君子湯

Used to treat early Ulgwang syndrome (Congestive-Hyperpsychotic syndrome), yang brightness syndrome, and excessiveness in the stomach-intestines.

人蔘 Ginseng Radix 7.5g
黃芪 Astragali Radix 3.75g
白朮 Atractylodis Rhizoma Alba 3.75g
白芍藥 Paeoniae Radix Alba 3.75g
當歸 Angelicae Gigantis Radix 3.75g
川芎 Cnidii Rhizoma 3.75g
陳皮 Citri Unshius Pericarpium 3.75g
炙甘草 Glycyrrhizae Radix et Rhizoma (stir-bake) 3.75g
生薑 Zingiberis Rhizoma Crudus 3 slices
大棗 Zizyphi Fructus 2 pulps

When 人蔘 Ginseng Radix is changed into 白何首烏 Cynanchi Wilfordii Radix, it is called SE14 Baekhaogunja-tang 白何烏君子湯 Cynanchi Wilfordii Radix Noble Decoction.
When 3.75g of 人蔘 Ginseng Radix is reduced, and 白何首烏 Cynanchi Wilfordii Radix and 官桂 Cinnamomi Cortex is added, it is called SE15 Sipjeondaebo-tang 十全大補湯 Ten Wholesome Greatly Tonifying Decoction.
When 37.5g of 人蔘 Ginseng Radix is used in this prescription, it is called SE16 Doksampalmul-tang 獨蔘八物湯 Ginseng-Emphasized Eight-Element Decoction.
When 黃芪 Astragali Radix is doubled and 官桂 Cinnamomi Cortex is changed into 陳皮 Citri Unshius Pericarpium, it is called SE17 Seungyangpalmul-tang 升陽八物湯 Yang-Upraising Eight-Element Decoction.
These 4 prescriptions are used to treat progressive syndrome of greater yang and yang brightness.

SE18 Cyperi Rhizoma Eight-Element Decoction
Hyangbujapalmul-tang 香附子八物湯

Used to treat damage in the spleen caused by worries, dry throat and tongue, and dull headache.

香附子 Cyperi Rhizoma 7.5g
當歸 Angelicae Gigantis Radix 7.5g
白芍藥 Paeoniae Radix Alba 7.5g
白朮 Atractylodis Rhizoma Alba 3.75g
白何烏 Polygoni Multiflori Radix Alba 3.75g
川芎 Cnidii Rhizoma 3.75g
陳皮 Citri Unshius Pericarpium 3.75g
炙甘草 Glycyrrhizae Radix et Rhizoma (stir-bake) 3.75g

When 3.75g of 乾薑 Zingiberis Rhizoma and 3.75g of 桂皮 Cinnamomi cortex are added; 3.75g of 當歸 Angelicae Gigantis Radix and 3.75g of 白芍藥 Paeoniae Radix Alba are reduced, it is called SE19 Hyangbusipjeon-tang 香附十全湯 Cyperi Rhizoma Ten Wholesome Decoction.

To treat stagnation syndrome and profuse sweating due to qi deficiency, change 香附子 Cyperi Rhizoma into 3.75g of 炮附子 Aconiti Lateralis Radix Preparata (stir-bake), and 生薑 Zingiberis Rhizoma Crudus 3 slices into 乾薑 Zingiberis Rhizoma.

10) The ingredients of this prescription is on SE92.

SE20 Cinnamomi, Pinelliae, and Zingiberis Decoction
Gyejibanhasaenggang-tang 桂枝半夏生薑湯

Used to treat vomiting due to deficiency cold and chest bind syndrome.

生薑 Zingiberis Rhizoma Crudus 11.25g
桂枝 Cinnamomi Ramulus 7.5g
半夏 Pinelliae Tuber 7.5g
白芍藥 Paeoniae Radix Alba 3.75g
白朮 Atractylodis Rhizoma Alba 3.75g
陳皮 Citri Unshius Pericarpium 3.75g
炙甘草 Glycyrrhizae Radix et Rhizoma (stir-bake) 3.75g

When 3.75g of 枳殼 Aurantii Fructus Immaturus, 靑皮 Citri Unshius Pericarpium Immaturus, 天南星 Arisaematis Rhizoma are added, it is called SE21 Geopung-san 祛風散 Wind-Dispelling Powder.

SE22 Cyperi Rhizoma and Amomi Fructus Stomach-Nourishing Decoction
Hyangsayangwi-tang 香砂養胃湯

Used to treat aversion to cold in the large intestine, yang brightness syndrome or excessiveness in the stomach-intestines, greater yin syndrome, food stagnation due to weak stomach, and jaundice.

人蔘 Ginseng Radix 3.75g
白朮 Atractylodis Rhizoma Alba 3.75g
白芍藥 Paeoniae Radix Alba 3.75g
炙甘草 Glycyrrhizae Radix et Rhizoma (stir-bake) 3.75g
半夏 Pinelliae Tuber 3.75g
香附子 Cyperi Rhizoma 3.75g
陳皮 Citri Unshius Pericarpium 3.75g
乾薑 Zingiberis Rhizoma 3.75g
山査肉 Crataegi Fructus 3.75g
砂仁 Amomi Fructus 3.75g
白荳蔲 Amomi Fructus Rotundus 3.75g

To treat dysentery, add 藿香 Agastachis Herba.

SE23 Polygoni Multiflori Radix and Cynanchi Wilfordii Radix Middle-Soothing Decoction
Jeokbaekhaogwanjung-tang 赤白何烏寬中湯

Used to treat patients experiencing exhaustion in all four limbs, difficult urination, impotency and the strong possibility of puffy swelling.

白何烏 Cynanchi Wilfordii Radix 3.75g
赤何烏 Polygoni Multiflori Radix 3.75g
良薑 Alpiniae Officinari Rhizoma 3.75g
乾薑 Zingiberis Rhizoma 3.75g
陳皮 Citri Unshius Pericarpium 3.75g
靑皮 Citri Unshius Pericarpium Immaturus 3.75g
香附子 Cyperi Rhizoma 3.75g
大棗 Zizyphi Fructus 2 pulps
益智仁 Alpiniae Oxyphyllae Fructus 3.75g

When 1.875g of 厚朴 Magnoliae Cortex, 1.875g of 枳實 Ponciri Fructus Immaturus, 1.875 of 木香 Aucklandiae Radix, 1.875g of 大腹皮 Arecae Pericarpium are added, it is called SE24 Sibimigwanjung-tang 十二味寬中湯 Twelve-Flavor Middle-Soothing Decoction.

To treat puffy swelling, 人蔘 Ginseng Radix should be changed into 赤何烏 Polygoni Multiflori Radix Rubra. It is called SE25 Insambaekhaogwanjung-tang 人蔘白何烏寬中湯 Ginseng Radix and Cynanchi Wilfordii Radix Middle-Soothing Decoction.

When 赤何烏 Polygoni Multiflori Radix Rubra is changed into 當歸 Angelicae Gigantis Radix, it is called SE26 Dangguibaekhaogwanjung-tang 當歸白何烏寬中湯 Angelicae Gigantis Radix and Cynanchi Wilfordii Radix Middle-Soothing Decoction.

When 3.75g of 五靈脂 Trogopterorum Faeces, and 3.75g of 益智仁 Alpiniae Oxyphyllae Fructus are added, this prescription can treat abdominal pain. It is called SE27 Oryeongjigwanjung-tang 五靈脂寬中湯 Trogopterorum Faeces Middle-Soothing Decoction.

When 白朮 Atractylodis Rhizoma Alba is added, it is called SE28 Gangchulgwanjung- tang 薑朮寬中湯 Zingiberis Rhizoma and Atractylodis Rhizoma Alba Middle-Soothing Decoction.

SE29 Allii Bulbus and Mel Paste
Sanmil-tang 蒜蜜湯

Used to treat dysentery.

白何烏 Polygoni Multiflori Radix Alba 3.75g
白朮 Atractylodis Rhizoma Alba 3.75g
白芍藥 Paeoniae Radix Alba 3.75g
桂枝 Cinnamomi Ramulus 3.75g
茵陳 Artemisiae Capillaris Herba 3.75g
益母草 Leonuri Herba 3.75g
赤石脂 Halloysitum Rubrum 3.75g
罌粟亮 Papaveris Fructus Deseminatus 3.75g
生薑 Zingiberis Rhizoma Crudus 3 slices
大棗 Zizyphi Fructus 2 pulps
大蒜 Alli Bulbus 5 roots
蜜 Mel a half spoonful

SE30 Chicken and Ginseng Radix Paste
Gyesam-go 鷄蔘膏

Used treat malaria and dysentery miraculously.

人蔘 Ginseng Radix 37.5g
桂皮 Cinnamomi Cortex 3.75g
鷄 Chicken 1

Stew and take the decoction.
If the patient has chronic malaria, first use 3.75g of 巴豆 Crotonis Semen as a purgative drug, and then take 鷄蔘膏 Chicken and Ginseng Radix Paste for several days. It also cure chronic malaria.

SE31 Crotonis Semen Pellet[11] Padu-dan 巴豆丹

巴豆(去殼) Crotonis Semen (remove husk) 1 kernel
Take this prescription with warm water.
If 巴豆 Crotonis Semen is stir-baked, it is called SE32 Onhwa-dan 溫化丹 Warming and Transforming Pellet.

SE33 Ginseng Radix and Citri Pericarpium Decoction Insamjinpi-tang 人蔘陳皮湯

Used to treat chronic infantile convulsions due to yin toxin. Take this prescription continuously for several days.

人蔘 Ginseng Radix 3.75g
生薑 Zingiberis Rhizoma Crudus 3.75g
砂仁 Amomi Fructus 3.75g
陳皮 Citri Unshius Pericarpium 3.75g

When 炮乾薑 Zingiberis Rhizoma (stir-bake) is substituted for 生薑 Zingiberis Rhizoma Crudus and 3.75g of Cinnamomi Cortex is added, it is called SE34 Insamgyepi-tang 人蔘桂皮湯 Ginseng Radix and Cinnamomi Cortex Decoction.

SE35 Ginseng Radix and Evodiae Fructus Decoction Insamosuyu-tang 人蔘吳茱萸湯

Used to treat greater yin and reverting yin syndrome.

人蔘 Ginseng Radix 37.5g
吳茱萸 Evodiae Fructus 11.25g
生薑 Zingiberis Rhizoma Crudus 11.25g
白芍藥 Paeoniae Radix Alba 3.75g
當歸 Angelicae Gigantis Radix 3.75g
蠐螬 Holotrichia Vermis 3.75g

11) There is no mention about efficacy of this prescription in the original text. Dongeisusebowon saids, "This will clear the contents in the stomach and intestines and raise the normal qi. After defecation, take Crotonis Semen continuously. A whole grain can induce diarrhea, while a half-grain can eliminate retained stool."

SE36

Cinnamomi Cortex and Aconiti Lateralis Preparata Radix Middle-Regulating Decoction

Bujaijung-tang 附子理中湯

It is also called Insambujagwangye-tang 人蔘附子官桂湯 Ginseng, Aconiti, and Cinnamomi Cortex Decoction.

人蔘 Ginseng Radix 11.25g
白朮 Atractylodis Rhizoma Alba 7.5g
乾薑(炮) Zingiberis Rhizoma (stir-bake) 7.5g
官桂 Cinnamomi Cortex 7.5g
白芍藥 Paeoniae Radix Alba 3.75g
陳皮 Citri Unshius Pericarpium 3.75g
炙甘草 Glycyrrhizae Radix et Rhizoma (stir-bake) 3.75g
附子(炮) Aconiti Lateralis Radix Preparata 3.75 or 7.5g

When 附子 Aconiti Lateralis Radix Preparata is removed and 18.75g of 人蔘 Ginseng Radix is added, it is called SE37 Doksamgwangyeijung-tang 獨蔘官桂理中湯 Ginseng-Emphasized Cinnamomi Cortex Middle-Regulating Decoction.
When 藿香 Agastachis Herba and 砂仁 Amomi Fructus are added, it is called SE38 Gyebugwakjinijung-tang 桂附藿陳理中湯 Cinnamomi, Aconiti, Agastachis, and Citri Unshius Middle-Regulating Decoction.
When 川芎 Cnidii Rhizoma, 當歸 Angelicae Gigantis Radix, 葱白 Allii Fistulosi Bulbus Fistular Onion Stalk, and 蘇葉 Perillae Folium, it is called SE39 Gungguichongsoijung-tang 芎歸葱蘇理中湯 Cnidii, Angelicae Gigantis, Allii Fistulosi, and Perillae Middle-Regulating Decoction.
Used to treat yin toxin disease due to greater yin syndrome.

- dry cholera
- visceral syncope
- yin exuberance with yang deficiency
- throat syndrome
- critical sign in greater and lesser yin syndrome

SE40

Evodiae Fructus and Aconiti Lateralis Radix Preparata Middle-Regulating Decoction

Osuyubujaijung-tang 吳茱萸附子理中湯

Used to treat visceral syncope, yin exuberance with yang blockage.

人蔘 Ginseng Radix 3.75g
白朮 Atractylodis Rhizoma Alba 3.75g
乾薑(炮) Zingiberis Rhizoma (stir-bake) 3.75g
官桂 Cinnamomi Cortex 3.75g
白芍藥 Paeoniae Radix Alba 3.75g
陳皮 Citri Unshius Pericarpium 3.75g
吳茱萸 Evodiae Fructus 3.75g
炙甘草 Glycyrrhizae Radix et Rhizoma (stir-bake) 3.75g
小茴香 Foeniculi Fructus 3.75g
補骨脂 Psoraleae Semen 3.75g
附子(炮) Aconiti Lateralis Radix Preparata (stir-bake) 3.75 or 7.5g

When 肉豆蔻(去油) Myristicae Semen (remove oil) is added, it is called SE41 Yukdugubujaijung-tang 肉豆久附子理中湯 Myristicae Semen and Aconiti Lateralis Radix Preparata Middle-Regulating Decoction.
This prescription is used to treat severe greater and lesser yin syndrome. Take 20 or 30 packs of this prescription continuously.

SE42 Cynanchi Wilfordii Radix and Aconiti Lateralis Radix Preparata Middle-Regulating Decoction Baekhaobujaijung-tang 白何烏附子理中湯

Used to treat greater yin syndrome; vomiting of roundworm due to stomach-cold.

白何首烏 Cynanchi Wilfordii Radix 11.25g
白朮(炒) Atractylodis Rhizoma Alba (stir-bake) 11.25g
白芍藥(炒) Paeoniae Radix Alba (stir-bake) 11.25g
桂枝 Cinnamomi Rhizoma 11.25g
乾薑(炮) Zingiberis Rhizoma 11.25g
陳皮 Citri Unshius Pericarpium 3.75g
附子 Aconiti Lateralis Radix Preparata 3.75g
甘草灸 Glycyrrhizae Radix et Rhizoma Preparata 3.75g

When 附子 Aconiti Lateralis Radix Preparata is removed, it is called SE43 Baekhaoijung-tang 白何烏理中湯 Cynanchi Wilfordii Radix Middle-Regulating Decoction.
When 7.5g of 大蒜 Alli Bulbus and 3.75g of 山査 Crataegi Fructus are added, it is called SE44 Sambaekijung-tang 三白理中湯 Three White Middle-Regulating Decoction.
Used to treat diarrhea due to internal damage.

SE45 Middle-Soothing Decoction Gwanjung-tang 寬中湯

Used to treat pain in the chest and abdomen.

乾薑 Zingiberis Rhizoma 3.75g
良薑 Alpiniae Officinari Rhizoma 3.75g
五靈脂 Trogopterorum Facecs 3.75g
益智仁 Alpiniae Oxyphyllae Fructus 3.75g
靑皮 Citri Unshius Pericarpium Immaturus 3.75g

SE46 Cinnamomi Ramulus Decoction Gyeji-tang 桂枝湯

桂枝 Cinnamomi Ramulus 11.25g
白芍藥 Paeoniae Radix Alba 7.5g
甘草 Glycyrrhizae Radix et Rhizoma 3.75g
大棗 Zizyphi Fructus 2 pulps
生薑 Zingiberis Rhizoma Crudus 3 slices

SE47 Middle-Regulating Decoction Ijung-tang 理中湯

人蔘 Ginseng Radix 7.5g
白朮 Atractylodis Rhizoma Alba 3.75g
乾薑 Zingiberis Rhizoma 3.75g
甘草炙 Glycyrrhizae Radix et Rhizoma Preparata 3.75g

When 陳皮 Citri Unshius Pericarpium, 官桂 Cinnamomi Cortex and 白何首烏 Polygoni Multiflori Radix Alba are added, it is called SE48 Baekhaogwangyeijung-tang 何烏官桂理中湯 Cynanchi Wilfordii Radi and Cinnamomi Cortex Middle-Regulating Decoction.

SE49 Gingiberis Rhizoma and Aconiti Lateralis Radix Preparata Decoction Gangbu-tang 薑附湯

乾薑炮 Zingiberis Rhizoma (stir-bake) 37.5g
附子炮 Aconiti Lateralis Radix Preparata 1 unit

Take this prescription boiled in water.

SE50 Four Counterflow Decoction Sayeok-tang 四逆湯

甘草炙 Glycyrrhizae Radix et Rhizoma Preparata 22.5g
乾薑炮 Zingiberis Rhizoma (stir-bake) 18.75g
生附子 Aconiti Lateralis Radix 1 unit

Grate the above drugs and take 2 packs decocted with water.

SE51 Halloysitum Rubrum and Limonitum Cum Terra Decoction
Jeokseokjiuyeoryang-tang 赤石脂禹餘粮湯

赤石脂 Halloysitum Rubrum 9.375g
禹餘粮 Limonitum Cum Terra 9.375g

SE52 Greatly Tonifying Decoction
Daebo-tang 大補湯

Used to treat consumptive disease.

人蔘 Ginseng Radix 3.75g
白朮 Atractylodis Rhizoma Alba 3.75g
白芍藥 Paeoniae Radix Alba 3.75g
甘草 Glycyrrhizae Radix et Rhizoma 3.75g
黃芪 Astragali Radix 3.75g
肉桂 Cinnamomi Cortex 3.75g
當歸 Angelicae Gigantis Radix 3.75g
川芎 Cnidii Rhizoma 3.75g
砂仁 Amomi Fructus 3.75g
陳皮 Citri Unshius Pericarpium 3.75g
生薑 Zingiberis Rhizoma Crudus 3 slices
大棗 Zizyphi Fructus 2 pulps

When 砂仁 Amomi Fructus and 陳皮 Citri Unshius Pericarpium are removed, and 3.75g of 乾薑 Zingiberis Rhizoma is added, it is called SE53 Hoeyangdaebo-tang 回陽大補湯 Yang-Restoring Greatly Tonifying Decoction.

SE54 Aucklandiae Radix Qi-Arranging Powder
Mokhyangsungi-san 木香順氣散

Used to treat qi stroke disease, suddenly violent angry due to qi counterflow and dizziness.

烏藥 Linderae Radix 3.75g
香附子 Cyperi Rhizoma 3.75g
青皮 Citri Unshius Pericarpium Immaturus 3.75g
陳皮 Citri Unshius Pericarpium 3.75g
厚朴 Magnoliae Cortex 3.75g
只殼 Aurantii Fructus Immaturus 3.75g
半夏 Pinelliae Tuber 3.75g
木香 Aucklandiae Radix 1.875g
縮砂 Amomi Fructus 1.875g
桂皮 Cinnamomi Rhizoma 1.125g
乾薑 Zingiberis Rhizoma 1.125g
甘草炙 Glycyrrhizae Radix et Rhizoma Preparata 1.125g
生薑 Zingiberis Rhizoma Crudus 3 slices
大棗 Zizyphi Fructus 2 pulps

SE55 Styrax Liquides Pill
Sohaphyang-won 蘇合香元

Used to treat all symptoms due to qi phlegm, qi stroke, qi ascent, qi counterflow, and qi pain.

白朮 Atractylodis Rhizoma Alba 75g
木香 Aucklandiae Radix 75g
沉香 Aquilariae Lignum 75g
丁香 Syzygii Flos 75g
安息香 Benzoinum 75g
白丹香 Santali Albi Lignum 75g
訶子肉 Chubulae Fructus 75g
香附子 Cyperi Rhizoma 75g
畢撥 Piperis Longi Fructus 75g
藿香 Agastachis Herba 75g
茴香 Foeniculi Fructus 75g
桂皮 Cinnamomi Cortex 75g
五靈脂 Trogopterorum Faeces 37.5g
玄胡索 Corydalis Tuber 37.5g

Make the above drugs into powder and mix them with the Benzoinum paste and honey. Pound 1000 times in a mortar. Make 40 boli from 37.5g of the resulting mixture. Two or three boli should be taken with spring water or warm water.

SE56 Cyperi Rhizoma and Perillae Folium Powder
Hyangso-san 香蘇散

Used to treat seasonal pestilence.

香附子 Cyperi Rhizoma 11.25g
蘇葉 Perillae Folium 9.375g
陳皮 Citri Unshius Pericarpium 3.75g
蒼术 Atractylodis Rhizoma 3.75g
甘草 Glycyrrhizae Radix et Rhizoma 3.75g
生薑 Zingiberis Rhizoma Crudus 3 slices
大棗 Zizyphi Fructus 2 pulps
蔥 Allii Fistulosi Bulbus 2 roots

SE57 Cinnamomi Ramulus and Aconiti Lateralis Radix Preparata Decoction
Gyejibuja-tang 桂枝附子湯

Used to treat leaking sweat and contracture of the limbs.

附子炮 Aconiti Lateralis Radix Preparata 11.25g
桂枝 Cinnamomi Ramulus 11.25g
白芍藥 Paeoniae Radix Alba 7.5g
甘草灸 Glycyrrhizae Radix et Rhizoma Preparata 3.75g

SE58 Artemisiae Capillaris Herba Four Counterflow Decoction
Injinsayeok-tang 茵陳四逆湯

Used to treat yin jaundice, and incessant cold sweating.

茵陳 Artemisiae Capillaris Herba 37.5g
附子炮 Aconiti Lateralis Radix Preparata 3.75g
乾薑炮 Zingiberis Rhizoma (bake) 3.75g
甘草灸 Glycyrrhizae Radix et Rhizoma Preparata 3.75g

When 乾薑 Zingiberis Rhizoma is removed, it is called SE59 Injinbuja-tang 茵陳附子湯 Artemisiae Capillaris Herba and Aconiti Lateralis Radix Preparata Decoction.
This prescription is used to treat yin jaundice and cold body.

SE60 Artemisiae Capillaris Herba and Citrus Unshius Pericarpium Decoction
Injingyulpi-tang 茵陳橘皮湯

Used to treat yin jaundice, and incessant panting and retching.

茵陳 Artemisiae Capillaris Herba 37.5g
陳皮 Citri Unshius Pericarpium 3.75g
白朮 Atractylodis Rhizoma Alba 3.75g
半夏 Pinelliae Tuber 3.75g
生薑 Zingiberis Rhizoma Crudus 3.75g

SE61 Three-Flavor Ginseng Radix and Evodiae Fructus Decoction
Sammisamyu-tang 三味蔘萸湯

Used to treat syncope, vomiting and drool foaming, lesser yin syndrome; agitation, yang brightness syndrome; desire to retch after eating.

吳茱萸 Evodiae Fructus 11.25g
人蔘 Ginseng Radix 7.5g
生薑 Zingiberis Rhizoma Crudus 3 slices
大棗 Zizyphi Fructus 2 pulps

SE62 Three-Flavor Ginseng Radix and Evodiae Fructus Decoction
Byeokryeok-san 霹靂散

附子炮 一個 Aconiti Lateralis Radix Preparata 1 unit

Decoct and remove the dregs, add honey and take it when it cools down. After a short time, the patient's irritability will cease, and he will perspire and fall asleep. Recovery follows.

SE63 White-Warming Pill
Onbaek-won 溫白元

Used to treat aggregation-accumulation, paraumbilical and hypochondriac aggregation, jaundice, tympanites, ten kinds of water qi, nine kinds of heart pain, eight kinds of glomus blockage, five kinds of numbness, and lingering malaria.

川烏炮 Aconiti Tuber (blast-bake) 93.75g
吳茱萸 Evodiae Fructus 18.75g
乾薑 Zingiberis Rhizoma 18.75g
肉桂 Cinnamomi Cortex 18.75g
川椒 Rubiae Radix 18.75g
赤伏苓 Poria (red) 18.75g
厚朴 Magnoliae Cortex 18.75g
人蔘 Ginseng Radix 18.75g
巴豆霜 Crotonis Semenis Pulvis 18.75g

Pulverize the above drugs and make pills with honey as big as a seed of a paulownia. Take three to seven pills with a decoction of Zingiberis Rhizoma Crudus 生薑.

SE64 Miasmic Jaundice Decoction
Jangdal-hwan 瘴疸丸

Used to treat seasonal pestilence.
• Endemic malaria, jaundice and dampness- heat disease.

茵陳 Artemisiae Capillaris Herba 37.5g
常山 Dichroae Radix 15g
鱉甲 Trionycis Carapax 15g
巴豆霜 Crotonis Semenis Pulvis 15g

Pulverize the drugs and make the pills as big as a seed of a paulownia. Take three to five pills with warm water.

SE65 Sparganii Rhizoma Accumulation-Dissolving Pill
Samneungsojeok-hwan 三稜消積丸

Used to treat indigestion induced by raw and cold food.

三稜 Sparganii Rhizoma 26.25g
蓬朮 Zedoariae Rhizoma 26.25g
神曲 Massa Medicata Fermentata 26.25g
巴豆(炒黑) Crotonis Semen (stir-bake to black) 18.75g
陳皮 Citri Unshius Pericarpium 18.75g
靑皮 Citri Unshius Pericarpium Immaturus 18.75g
茴香 Foeniculi Fructus 18.75g
丁香皮 Caryophylli Flos 11.25g
益智仁 Alpiniae Oxyphyllae Fructus 11.25g

Make the pasted pills with vinegar as big as a seed of a paulownia. Take 30-40 pills with the decoction of 生薑 Zingiberis Rhizoma Crudus.

SE66 Secret Stagnation-Harmonizing Pill Bibanghwache-hwan 秘方和滯丸

Used to treat seasonal pestilence.

• Endemic malaria, jaundice and dampness- heat disease.

三稜 Sparganii Rhizoma 15g
蓬朮(煨) Zedoariae Rhizoma (roast) 15g
半夏 Pinelliae Tuber 9.375g
木香 Aucklandiae Radix 9.375g
丁香 Syzygii Flos 9.375g
陳皮 Citri Unshius Pericarpium 9.375g
靑皮 Citri Unshius Pericarpium Immaturus 9.375g
黃連 Coptidis Rhizoma 9.375g
巴豆(醋浸一宿) Crotonis Semen (steep in vinegar for one night) 22.5g

Pulverize the above drugs with 烏梅 Mume Fructus and some wheat flour. And make paste pills as big as an oat. Take five to ten pills. In order to facilitate bowel movement, take with hot water. To purge the bowels, take with cold water. Harmonization comes from clearing blockage; regulatig yin and yang comes from supplementation and drainage.

SE67 Three-Element White Powder Sammulbaek-san 三物白散

桔梗 Platycodonis Radix 11.25g
貝母 Fritillariae Cirrhosae Bulbus 11.25g
巴豆(熬研) Crotonis Semen (stew and grind) 3.75g

Pulverize the above drugs. Mix 1.875g of the drugs with hot water and have the patient take it. If the patient is weak, the dosage should be reduced by half. In case the patient vomits or has diarrhea, give a cup of hot rice gruel. In case of ceaseless diarrhea, a cup of cold rice gruel should be given.

SE68 Pliant Pellet Yeoui-dan 如意丹

Used to treat pestilence, possessedness, forest miasmic qi, mania and withdrawal, loss of mind, yin and yang two toxin, five malaria, five malnutrition, eight dysentery, and failure to acclimatize to a new environment.

川烏炮 Aconiti Tuber (blast-bake) 30g
人蔘 Ginseng Radix 18.75g
吳茱萸 Evodiae Fructus 18.75g
川椒 Zanthoxyli Fructus 18.75g
白伏苓 Poria Sclerotium (white) 18.75g
白薑蠶 Batryticatus Bombyx 18.75g
厚朴 Magnoliae Cortex 18.75g
肉桂 Cinnamomi Cortex 18.75g
當歸 Angelicae Gigantis Radix 18.75g
巴豆霜 Crotonis Semenis Pulvis 9.375g

SE69 Cyperi Rhizoma and Amomi Fructus Six Noble Decoction Hyangsayukgunja-tang 香砂六君子湯

Used to treat loss of interest in food and drink, inability to get food and drink down, bloating after eating.

香附子 Cyperi Rhizoma 3.75g
白朮 Atractylodis Rhizoma Alba 3.75g
白伏苓 Poria Sclerotium (white) 3.75g
半夏 Pinelliae Tuber 3.75g
陳皮 Citri Unshius Pericarpium 3.75g
厚朴 Magnoliae Cortex 3.75g
白豆蔲 Amomi Fructus Rotundus 3.75g
人蔘 Ginseng Radix 1.875g
甘草 Glycyrrhizae Radix et Rhizoma 1.875g
木香 Aucklandiae Radix 1.875g
縮砂 Amomi Fructus 1.875g
益智仁 Alpiniae Oxyphyllae Fructus 1.875g
生薑 Zingiberis Rhizoma Crudus 3 slices
大棗 Zizyphi Fructus 2 pulps

SE70 Yin-Suppressing Tartare Jineum-hoe 鎭陰膾

Used to treat puffy swelling.

獐肝 Roe deer liver 1 unit

SE71 Life-Protecting Decoction Bomyeong-eum 保命飮

Used to treat puffy swelling.

海鹽 Sea salt

Extract juice and take a spoonful of it every time. And take it until the total amount of them becomes a cup.

SE72 Red-Colored Serpent Decoction Jeoksa-jeon 赤蛇煎

Used to treat dysentery.

項赤巳 Red-Colored Serpent

Remove head and tail. And put the rest into the double sack. Prepare a pot and hang the sack on the bar that crosses the mouth of the pot. Decoct it with 5 bowls of water until a bowl of water remains in the pot. Then take the contents of the sack. This is the method for removing poison of serpent's bone.

SE73 Garlic and Honey Paste Sanmil-go 蒜蜜膏

Used to treat dysentery.

大蒜 Allii Bulbus 3 units

清蜜 Mel half spoonful

SE74 Ginseng Radix Powder Insam-san 人蔘散

Used to treat all sores.

人蔘 Ginseng Radix

Pulverize the above drug and attach to an affected area.

SE75

Pliant Needle

Yeoui-chim 如意針

To effuse an abscess area, use fire needle and take pus.

火針 Fire needle

SE76

Pliant Blade

Yeoui-do 如意刀

Welling-abscess of the back should be cut open with a fire blade in the initial stages. If it should not be done, it becomes hardened and difficult to treat.

火刀 Fire Blade

SE77

Paralysis Decoction

Bulsu-eum 不遂飮

Used to treat hemiplegia.

鐵液水 Ferric Oxide

SE78

Middle warming Decoction

Onjung-eum 溫中飮

Used to treat food stagnation of pregnant women.

生薑 Zingiberis Rhizoma Crudus

Extract juice and take it.

SE79 Liver-Warming Powder Nangan-san 煖肝散

Use to treat eye disease and dim vision.

尾蔘 Ginseng Radix Palva
何烏 Polygoni Multiflori Radix

Pulverize the above drugs, and mix with honey water. Take this prescription until perspiration. And this prescription also can be used for an eye wash.

SE80 Sulfur Powder Yuhwang-san 硫黃散

Used to treat eye disease.
• Snake bite

硫黃 Sulfur

Pulverize the above drug and apply it to a paper. Then apply on the closed eye and let stand overnight.

SE81 Gold-Colored Serpent Liquor Geumsa-ju 金蛇酒

Used to treat sore throat.

金色黃章蛇 Gold-Colored Serpent

Make it liquor and drink.

SE82 Deviation-Correcting Powder
Gyeonjeong-san 牽正散

Used to treat deviation due to wind stroke.

白附子 Aconiti Koreani Tuber equal amount
白薑蠶 Batryticatus Bombyx equal amount
全蝎(生用) Scorpio (use in raw) equal amount

Take 7.5g of the prescription with wine.

SE83 Rubi Flos and Citri Fructus Preparata Decoction
Danggyul-tang 唐橘湯

Used to treat wind stroke with paralysis and hemiplegia.

橘餅 Citri Fructus Preparata 5 cups
唐花 Rubi Flos 1 handful

Boil this prescription in water and take in one single dose. Repeat this until recovery.

SE84 Spleen-Longevity Speech-Releasing Decoction
Subihaeeo-tang 壽脾解語湯

Used to treat wind stroke with loss of speech.

白何烏 Polygoni Multiflori Radix Alba equal amount
紫蘇葉 Perillae Folium equal amount
南星 Arisaematis Rhizoma equal amount
黃芪 Astragali Radix equal amount
桂枝 Cinnamomi Ramulus equal amount

SE85 Seven Qi Decoction
Chilgi-tang 七氣湯

Used to treat seven emotions binding depression.

半夏 Pinelliae Tuber 11.25g
人蔘 Ginseng Radix 2.625g
官桂 Cinnamomi Cortex 2.625g
甘草 Glycyrrhizae Radix et Rhizoma Preparata 2.625g

SE86 Qi-Correcting Linderae Radix and Cyperi Rhizoma Decoction
Jeonggicheonhyang-tang 正氣天香湯

Used to treat nine qi pain.

香附子 Cyperi Rhizoma 11.25g
烏藥 Linderae Radix 7.5g
陳皮 Citri Unshius Pericarpium 7.5g
蘇葉 Perillae Folium 7.5g
乾薑 Zingiberis Rhizoma 1.875g
甘草 Glycyrrhizae Radix et Rhizoma 1.875g

SE87 Citrus Unshiu Decoction
Gamgyul-jeon 甘橘煎

Used to promote lactation.

好橘 Citrus Unshiu of good quality 30 kernels
肥棗(蒸) Fat Zizyphi Fructus (steam) 1.8 L
陳粟米 Washing millet 1.8 L
當歸 Angelicae Gigantis Radix 600g
甘草 Glycyrrhizae Radix et Rhizoma 18.75g

Decoct honey and 葱 Alli Radix, and remove the dregs. Administer randomly.

SE88 Marvelous Decoction Yeosin-tang 如神湯

Used to treat lumbar pain.

玄胡索 Corydalis Tuber equal amount
當歸 Angelicae Gigantis Radix equal amount
香附子 Cyperi Rhizoma equal amount
桂心 Cassiae Cortex Interior equal amount
木香 Aucklandiae Radix equal amount

Pulverize the ingredients. Take 7.5g of the prescription with ginger water.

SE89 Crotonis Semen Paste Padu-go 巴豆膏

Used to treat all kinds of sores.

巴豆(去殼炒) Crotonis Semen (remove the shell and stir-bake)

Make paste and attach it to a lesion.

SE90 Eight-Element Added Decoction Gamipalmul-tang 加味八物湯

Used to treat fetal bleeding.

人蔘 Ginseng Radix 7.5g
當歸 Angelicae Gigantis Radix 7.5g
黃芪 Astragali Radix 7.5g
川芎 Cnidii Rhizoma 7.5g
白朮 Atractylodis Rhizoma Alba 3.75g
白芍藥 Paeoniae Radix Alba 3.75g
陳皮 Citri Unshius Pericarpium 3.75g
甘草 Glycyrrhizae Radix et Rhizoma Preparata 3.75g
香附子(炒) Cyperi Rhizoma (stir-bake) 3.75g
艾葉 Artemisiae Argyi Folium 7.5g
大棗 Zizyphi Fructus 20g

SE91 Agastachis Herba Qi-Correcting Powder Gwakhyangjeonggi-san 藿香正氣散

Used to treat greater yang pattern; aversion of cold in the large intestine.
- Yang brightness pattern; failing to release the exterior, greater yin pattern; clear food diarrhea.

藿香 Agastachis Herba 5.625g
紫蘇 Perillae Folium 3.75g
蒼朮 Atractylodis Rhizoma 1.875g
白朮 Atractylodis Rhizoma Alba 1.875g
半夏 Pinelliae Tuber 1.875g
陳皮 Citri Unshius Pericarpium 1.875g
大卜皮 Arecae Pericarpium 1.875g
靑皮 Citri Unshius Pericarpium Immaturus 1.875g
桂皮 Cinnamomi Cortex 1.875g
乾干 Zingiberis Rhizoma 1.875g
益智仁 Alpiniae Oxyphyllae Fructus 1.875g
灸甘草 Glycyrrhizae Radix et Rhizoma 1.875g

- To treat retention of the placenta, multiply 陳皮 Citri Unshius Pericarpium by five.
- When 木香 Aucklandiae Radix and 南星 Arisaematis Rhizoma are added, it is called SE92 Seonghyangjeonggi-san 星香正氣散 Arisaematis Rhizoma and Aucklandiae Radix Qi-Correcting Powder.

This prescription is used to treat wind stroke, qi stroke, phlegm syncope, crapulent syncope. Take this medicine first and choose treatment methods according to patterns.

SE93 Amomi Fructus Powder Sain-san 砂仁散

Used to treat mistakenly swallowing gold, silver, etc.

砂仁(研) Amomi Fructus (grind) 7.5 or 18.75g

Grind to a fine powder and take with warm water.

Empirical Prescriptions for Soeum Type 少陽人 經驗方

SE-e1 Astragali Radix and Perillae Folium Decoction Hwanggisoyeop-tang 黃芪蘇葉湯

Used to treat exterior fever, aversion to cold, and sweating. And also used to treat external contraction for 3-4 days.

黃芪 Astragali Radix 15g
桂枝 Cinnamomi Ramulus 7.5g
白芍藥 Paeoniae Radix Alba 7.5g
川芎 Cnidii Rhizoma 3.75g
當歸 Angelicae Gigantis Radix 3.75g
蘇葉 Perillae Folium 3.75g
甘草(炙) Glycyrrhizae Radix et Rhizoma Preparata 3.75g

SE-e2 Spleen-Fortifying Stomach-Strengthening Decoction Geonbijangwi-tang 健脾壯胃湯

Used to treat yang brightness disease; fever and copious sweat.
• Stomach cold, ascaris above the diaphragm.

人蔘 Ginseng Radix 3.75g
黃芪 Astragali Radix 3.75g
官桂 Cinnamomi Cortex 3.75g
當歸 Angelicae Gigantis Radix 3.75g
川芎 Cnidii Rhizoma 3.75g
白芍藥 Paeoniae Radix Alba 3.75g
甘草(炙) Glycyrrhizae Radix et Rhizoma Preparata 3.75g
乾薑 Zingiberis Rhizoma 3.75g
白朮 Atractylodis Rhizoma Alba 3.75g
陳皮 Citri Unshius Pericarpium 3.75g
蘇葉 Perillae Folium 1.875g
附子 Aconiti Lateralis Radix Preparata 1.875g
生薑 Zingiberis Rhizoma Crudus 3 slices
大棗 Zizyphi Fructus 2 pulps

SE-e3 Tonifying-Replenishing Qi-Securing Decoction Boikgogi-tang 補益固氣湯

Used to treat yang brightness pattern; aversion to heat rather than cold, and sweating.

黃芪 Astragali Radix 7.5g
桂枝 Cinnamomi Ramulus 7.5g
人蔘 Ginseng Radix 7.5g
白芍藥 Paeoniae Radix Alba 3.75g
甘草(炙) Glycyrrhizae Radix et Rhizoma Preparata 3.75g

當歸 Angelicae Gigantis Radix 3.75g
川芎 Cnidii Rhizoma 3.75g
白朮 Atractylodis Rhizoma Alba 3.75g
陳皮 Citri Unshius Pericarpium 3.75g

It is also good to add 3.75g of 官桂 Cinnamomi Cortex, 3.75g of 乾薑 Zingiberis Rhizoma, and 1.875g of 附子 Aconiti Lateralis Radix Preparata.

SE-e4 Cinnamomi Cortex Ginseng-Emphasized Eight-Element Decoction Gwangyedoksampalmul-tang 官桂獨蔘八物湯

Used to treat yang-brightness exterior pattern, fever and copious sweating.
• Also used to treat hematemesis.

人蔘 Ginseng Radix 18.75g
黃芪 Astragali Radix 11.25g
白朮 Atractylodis Rhizoma Alba 3.75g
白芍藥 Paeoniae Radix Alba 3.75g
當歸 Angelicae Gigantis Radix 3.75g
川芎 Cnidii Rhizoma 3.75g
官桂 Cinnamomi Cortex 3.75g
甘草(灸) Glycyrrhizae Radix et Rhizoma Preparata 3.75g

SE-e5 Atractylodis Rhizoma and Zingiberis Rhizoma Accumulation-Breaking Decoction Gangchulpajeok-tang 薑朮破積湯

Used to treat lower abdominal fullness, aversion to cold in the chest.
• Vomiting and diarrhea, stomach qi deficiency, food stagnation, yellow flat-abscess, and diarrhea with clear water.

蒼朮 Atractylodis Rhizoma 3.75g
白朮 Atractylodis Rhizoma Alba 3.75g
良薑 Alpiniae Officinari Rhizoma 3.75g
乾薑 Zingiberis Rhizoma 3.75g
何首烏 Polygoni Multiflori Radix 3.75g
大蒜 Allii Bulbus 3.75g
陳皮 Citri Unshius Pericarpium 3.75g
靑皮 Citri Unshius Pericarpium Immaturus 3.75g
厚朴 Magnoliae Cortex 3.75g
只實 Ponciri Fructus Immaturus 3.75g
木香 Aucklandiae Radix 3.75g
大腹皮 Arecae Pericarpium 3.75g
白芍藥 Paeoniae Radix Alba 1.875g
甘草(灸) Glycyrrhizae Radix et Rhizoma Preparata 1.875g

SE-e6

Agastachis Herba and Amomi Fructus Middle-Regulating Decoction

Hyangsaijung-tang 香砂理中湯

Used to treat diarrhea due to internal damage, abdominal fullness and vomiting, food stagnation and jaundice.

人蔘 Ginseng Radix 7.5g
白朮 Atractylodis Rhizoma Alba 7.5g
乾薑 Zingiberis Rhizoma 7.5g
白芍藥 Paeoniae Radix Alba 7.5g
砂仁 Amomi Fructus 3.75g
藿香 Agastachis Herba 3.75g
陳皮 Citri Unshius Pericarpium 3.75g
甘草(灸) Glycyrrhizae Radix et Rhizoma Preparata 3.75g
大棗 Zizyphi Fructus 2 pulps

SE-e7

Ginseng-Emphasized Middle-Regulating Decoction

Doksamijung-tang 獨蔘理中湯

Used to treat ascaris above the diaphragm due to stomach cold.

人蔘 Ginseng Radix 18.75g
白朮 Atractylodis Rhizoma Alba 7.5g
乾薑 Zingiberis Rhizoma 7.5g
白芍藥 Paeoniae Radix Alba 7.5g
陳皮 Citri Unshius Pericarpium 3.75g
甘草(灸) Glycyrrhizae Radix et Rhizoma Preparata 3.75g
大棗 Zizyphi Fructus 2 pulps

When 7.5g of 附子 Aconiti Lateralis Radix Preparata added, the efficiency of the medicine will get better.

SE-e8

Cinnamomi, Allii Fistulosi, and Perillae Middle-Regulating Decoction

Gyejichongsoijung-tang 桂枝葱蘇理中湯

Used to treat jaundice, smaller-abdominal fullness, diarrhea with clear water, and dry mouth.

人蔘 Ginseng Radix 7.5g
白朮 Atractylodis Rhizoma Alba 7.5g
白芍藥 Paeoniae Radix Alba 7.5g
乾薑 Zingiberis Rhizoma 3.75g
甘草(灸) Glycyrrhizae Radix et Rhizoma Preparata 3.75g
當歸 Angelicae Gigantis Radix 3.75g
附子 Aconiti Lateralis Radix Preparata 3.75g
川芎 Cnidii Rhizoma 3.75g
桂枝 Cinnamomi Ramulus 3.75g
蘇葉 Perillae Folium 3.75g
葱 Allii Fistulosi Bulbus 3 roots
大棗 Zizyphi Fructus 2 pulps

SE-e9 Ginseng Radix and Papaveris Fructus Deseminatus Decoction Insamaengsok-tang 人蔘罌粟湯

Used to treat dysentery.

人蔘 Ginseng Radix 3.75g
白朮 Atractylodis Rhizoma Alba 3.75g
白芍藥 Paeoniae Radix Alba 3.75g
益母草 Leonuri Herba 3.75g
陳皮 Citri Unshius Pericarpium 3.75g
罌粟殼 Papaveris Fructus Deseminatus 3.75g
甘草 Glycyrrhizae Radix et Rhizoma 3.75g

SE-e10 Ginseng-Emphasized Friendly Decoction Doksamyangbung-tang 獨蔘良朋湯

Used to treat infantile diarrhea, and chronic infantile convulsion.

人蔘 Ginseng Radix 37.5g
生薑 Zingiberis Rhizoma Crudus 7.5g
當歸 Angelicae Gigantis Radix 3.75g
官桂 Cinnamomi Cortex 3.75g
陳皮 Citri Unshius Pericarpium 3.75g
大棗 Zizyphi Fructus 2 pulps

SE-e11 Chicken and Astragali Radix Paste Gyegi-go 鷄芪膏

Used to treat malaria, and dysentery.

黃芪 Astragali Radix 37.5g
桂枝 Cinnamomi Ramulus 18.75g
鷄 1 Chicken

Stew and take the decoction.

SE-e12

Perillae Semen Phlegm-Conducting Decoction

Sojadodam-tang 蘇子導痰湯

Used to treat phlegm panting.

蘇子 Perillae Semen 7.5g
半夏 Pinelliae Tuber 5.625g
當歸 Angelicae Gigantis Radix 5.625g
南星 Arisaematis Rhizoma 3.75g
陳皮 Citri Unshius Pericarpium 3.75g
厚朴 Magnoliae Cortex 2.625g
只實 Ponciri Fructus Immaturus 2.625g
甘草 Glycyrrhizae Radix et Rhizoma 1.875g

SE-e13

Angelicae Gigantis Radix Middle-Warming Decoction

Dangguionjung-tang 當歸溫中湯

Used to treat internal damage of blood and qi.

當歸 Angelicae Gigantis Radix 11.25g
白芍藥 Paeoniae Radix Alba 9.375g
白何烏 Polygoni Multiflori Radix Alba 3.75g
白朮 Atractylodis Rhizoma Alba 3.75g
川芎 Cnidii Rhizoma 3.75g
桂枝 Cinnamomi Ramulus 3.75g
黃芪 Astragali Radix 3.75g
玄胡索 Corydalis Tuber 3.75g
益母草 Leonuri Herba 3.75g
生薑 Zingiberis Rhizoma Crudus 3 slices
大棗 Zizyphi Fructus 2 pulps

Soyang Type 少陽人

SY1

Schizonepetae Spica and Saposhnikoviae Radix Toxin-Repelling Powder

Hyeongbangpaedok-san 荊防敗毒散

Used to treat headache, alternation of cold and heat.

- Greater yang pattern
- Lesser yang pattern
- When there are sudden vomiting and tertian malaria, take 2 packs of this medicine decocted in advance at a time. It can be used by 20 packs.

羌活 Osterici Radix 3.75g
獨活 Angelicae Continentalis Radix 3.75g
柴胡 Bupleuri Radix 3.75g
前胡 Angelicae Decursivae Radix 3.75g
荊芥 Schizonepetae Spica 3.75g
防風 Saposhnikoviae Radix 3.75g
赤伏苓 Poria Sclerotium Rubra 3.75g
生地黃 Rehmanniae Radix Crudus 3.75g
車前子 Plantaginis Semen 3.75g

SY2

Schizonepetae Spica and Saposhnikoviae Radix Red-Conducting Powder

Hyeongbangdojeok-san 荊防導赤散

Used to treat lesser yang headache, chest bind, and agitation in the chest and diaphragm.

生地黃 Rehmanniae Radix Crudus 11.25g
木通 Akebiae Caulis 7.5g
玄蔘 Scrophulariae Radix 5.625g
苽蔞仁 Trichosanthis Semen 5.625g
前胡 Angelicae Decursivae Radix 3.75g
羌活 Osterici Radix 3.75g
獨活 Angelicae Continentalis Radix 3.75g
荊芥 Schizonepetae Spica 3.75g
防風 Saposhnikoviae Radix 3.75g

When 伏苓 Poria Sclerotium and 澤瀉 Alismatis Rhizoma are added, SY3 Dojeokganggi-tang 導赤降氣湯 Red-Conducting Qi-Lowering Decoction.

SY4 Schizonepetae Spica and Saposhnikoviae Radix White-Draining Powder Hyeongbangsabaek-san 荊防瀉白散

Used to treat headache, bladder pain, agitation, lesser yang pattern, generalized heat and headache, diarrhea, yin collapse syndrome.

生地黃 Rehmanniae Radix Crudus 11.25g
伏苓 Poria Sclerotium 7.5g
澤瀉 Gypsum Fibrosum 3.75g
知母 Anemarrhenae Rhizoma 3.75g
羌活 Osterici Radix 3.75g
荊芥 Schizonepetae Spica 3.75g
防風 Saposhnikoviae Radix 3.75g

When 黃連 Coptidis Rhizoma, 苽蔞仁 Trichosanthis Semen are added, it is called SY5 Hwangryeonsabaek-san 黃連瀉白散 Coptidis Rhizoma White-Draining Powder
Used to treat greater yang syndrome with stomach heat and interior heat, and constipation during a day.

SY6 Polyporus and Plantaginis Semen Decoction Jeoryeongchajeonja-tang 猪苓車前子湯

Used to treat fever and diarrhea due to yin collapse disease.
- Headache and abdominal pain due to yang brightness syndrome and triple yang combination disease.

澤瀉 Alismatis Rhizoma 7.5g
伏苓 Poria Sclerotium 7.5g
猪苓 Polyporus 5.625g
車前子 Plantaginis Semen 5.625g
知母 Anemarrhenae Rhizoma 3.75g
石膏 Gypsum Fibrosum 3.75g
羌活 Osterici Radix 3.75g
獨活 Angelicae Continentalis Radix 3.75g
荊芥 Schizonepetae Spica 3.75g
防風 Saposhnikoviae Radix 3.75g

SY7 Talcum and Sophorae Radix Decoction Hwalseokgosam-tang 滑石苦蔘湯

Used to treat yin collapse syndrome with abdominal pain and cold body but no diarrhea, and abdominal pain for 2,3 days or 4,5 times a day.

澤瀉 Alismatis Rhizoma 7.5g
伏苓 Poria Sclerotium 7.5g
滑石 Talcum 7.5g
苦蔘 Sophorae Radix 7.5g
川黃連 Coptidis Rhizoma 3.75g
黃栢 Phellodendri Cortex 3.75g
羌活 Osterici Radix 3.75g

Angelicae Pubescentis Radix and Rehmanniae Radix Preparata Decoction

SY8 Dokhwaljihwang-tang 獨活地黃湯

Used to treat stuffiness and fullness due to food stagnation.

- Cyclically rising heat in noon due to yin deficiency.
- Wind stroke with vomiting, and cold drool in the mouth. If there is counterflow qi ascent, it can also cause vomiting.
- When there is tertian malaria, take 2 packs of this medicine in the morning and evening. It can be used by 40 packs.
- Early stage of deviated eye and mouth.

熟地黃 Rehmanniae Radix Preparata 15g
山茱萸 Corni Fructus 7.5g
伏苓 Poria Sclerotium 5.625g
澤瀉 Alismatis Rhizoma 5.625g
牧丹皮 Moutan Cortex 3.75g
防風 Saposhnikoviae Radix 3.75g
獨活 Angelicae Continentalis Radix 3.75g

Schizonepetae, Saposhnikoviae, and Rehmanniae Radix Preparata Decoction

SY9 Hyeongbangjihwang-tang 荊防地黃湯

Used to treat cold body and diarrhea due to yin collapse syndrome.

- Puffy swelling from early stage to convalescence.
- 荊芥 Schizonepetae Spica, 防風 Saposhnikoviae Radix, 羌活 Osterici Radix, 獨活 Angelicae Continentalis Radix are al drugs nourishing yin. 荊芥 Schizonepetae Spica and 防風 Saposhnikoviae Radix are very effective in clearing away heat from the chest and dispelling the wind. 羌活 Osterici Radix and 獨活 Angelicae Continentalis Radix have the effect of greatly tonifying the genuine yin of the bladder. Whether he suffers from a headache, abdominal pain, a feeling of fullness in the chest and upper abdomen, or diarrhea, a weak patient taking hundreds of packs of this medicine will recover; it is very effective medicine.

熟地黃 Rehmanniae Radix Preparata 7.5g
山茱萸 Corni Fructus 7.5g
伏苓 Poria Sclerotium 7.5g
澤瀉 Alismatis Rhizoma 7.5g
車前子 Plantaginis Semen 3.75g
羌活 Osterici Radix 3.75g
獨活 Angelicae Continentalis Radix 3.75g
荊芥 Schizonepetae Spica 3.75g
防風 Saposhnikoviae Radix 3.75g

To treat cough, add 前胡 Angelicae Decursivae Radix. It is called SY10 Jeonhojihwang-tang 前胡地黃湯 Angelicae Decursivae Radix and Rehmanniae Radix Preparata Decoction.

To treat blood pattern, add 玄蔘 Scrophulariae Radix and 牧丹皮 Moutan Cortex. It is called SY11 Hyunsamjihwang-tang 玄蔘地黃湯 Scrophulariae Radix and Rehmanniae Radix Preparata Decoction.
To treat hemilateral headache, add 黃連 Coptidis Rhizoma and 牛蒡子 Arctii Fructus. It is called SY12 Hwangryeonjihwang-tang 黃連地黃湯 Coptidis Rhizoma and Rehmanniae Radix Preparata Decoction.
To treat stuffiness and fullness due to food stagnation, add 牧丹皮 Moutan Cortex. It is called SY13 Mokdanjihwang-tang 牧丹地黃湯 Moutan Cortex and Rehmanniae Radix Preparata Decoction.
To treat fire pattern, remove 山茱萸 Corni Fructus and add 石膏 Gypsum Fibrosum. It is called SY14 Ganghwajihwang-tang 降火地黃湯 Fire-Lowering Rehmanniae Radix Preparata Decoction.
To treat headache, vexing heat, and blood pattern, use 生地黃 Rehmanniae Radix Crudus. It is called SY15 Saengsukjihwang-tang 生熟地黃湯 Rehmanniae Radix Crudus et Preparata Decoction.
To treat puffy swelling, add 11.25g of 木通 Akebiae Caulis. It is called SY16 Moktongmuwu-tang 木通無憂湯 Akebiae Caulis Anxiety-Free Decoction.

SY17 Twelve-Flavor Rehmanniae Radix Preparata Decoction
Sibimijihwang-tang 十二味地黃湯

Used to treat blood ejection, cyclically rising heat in noon due to yin deficiency.
- Genital disease
- Epilepsy
- This prescription is also called Sibimiguisin-tang 十二味歸腎湯 Twelve-Flavor Kidney-Restoring Decoction.

熟地黃 Rehmanniae Radix Preparata 15g
山茱萸 Corni Fructus 11.25g
白伏苓 Poria Sclerotium Alba 7.5g
澤瀉 Alismatis Rhizoma 7.5g
牧丹皮 Moutan Cortex 3.75g
地骨皮 Lycii Cortex 3.75g
玄蔘 Scrophulariae Radix 3.75g
枸杞子 Lycii Fructus 3.75g
覆盆子 Rubi Fructus 3.75g
車前子 Plantaginis Semen 3.75g
荊芥 Schizonepetae Spica 3.75g
防風 Saposhnikoviae Radix 3.75g

SY18 Rehmanniae Radix Crudus White Tiger Decoction
Jihwangbaekho-tang 地黃白虎湯

Used to treat chest bind, delirious speech.

- Yin collapse; delirious speech, greater yang pattern similar to malaria.
- Yang brightness pattern; agitation, constipation.
- Interior heat, rough stool. Irrespectively of interior or exterior, this prescription should be used to treat constipation, and also used to treat delirious speech.
- This prescription is also used to treat flailing of arms and legs, taking fluids, mania, curled tongue stirring wind.

石膏 Gypsum Fibrosum 18.75 or 37.5g
生地黃 Rehmanniae Radix Crudus 15g
知母 Anemarrhenae Rhizoma 7.5g
防風 Saposhnikoviae Radix 3.75g
獨活 Angelicae Continentalis Radix 3.75g

SY19 Yang Toxin White Tiger Decoction Yangdokbaekho-tang 陽毒白虎湯

Used to treat yang toxin macular eruption and fecal block.

- Throat-entwining wind
- Swollen lips
- To treat stirring wind, adding 3.75g of 羌活 Osterici Radix and 獨活 Angelicae Continentalis Radix, 1.875g of 柴胡 Bupleuri Radix, 玄蔘 Scrophulariae Radix, 山梔子 Gardeniae Fructus, 忍冬 Lonicerae Folium et Caulis, and 薄荷 Menthae Herba is more wonderful.

石膏 Gypsum Fibrosum 18.75 or 37.5g
生地黃 Rehmanniae Radix Crudus 15g
知母 Anemarrhenae Rhizoma 7.5g
荊芥 Schizonepetae Spica 3.75g
防風 Saposhnikoviae Radix 3.75g
牛蒡子 Arctii Fructus 3.75g

SY20 Diaphragm-Cooling Fire-Dissipating Decoction Yanggyeoksanhwa-tang 凉膈散火湯

Used to treat upper wasting-thirst, throat-entwining wind and mild pattern of swollen lips.

生地黃 Rehmanniae Radix Crudus 7.5g
忍冬藤 Lonicerae Folium et Caulis 7.5g
連翹 Forsythiae Fructus 7.5g
山梔子 Gardeniae Fructus 3.75g
薄荷 Menthae Herba 3.75g
知母 Anemarrhenae Rhizoma 3.75g
石膏 Gypsum Fibrosum 3.75g
防風 Saposhnikoviae Radix 3.75g
荊芥 Schizonepetae Spica 3.75g

SY21 Lonicerae Caulis and Lycii Radicis Cortex Decoction
Indongdeungjigolpi-tang 忍冬藤地骨皮湯

Used to treat cold body, abdominal pain, and diarrhea.

忍冬藤 Lonicerae Caulis 15g
地骨皮 Lycii Radicis Cortex 7.5g
山茱萸 Corni Fructus 7.5g
川黃連 Coptidis Rhizoma 3.75g
黃栢 Phellodendri Cortex 3.75g
玄蔘 Scrophulariae Radix 3.75g
苦蔘 Sophorae Radix 3.75g
生地黃 Rehmanniae Radix Crudus 3.75g
知母 Anemarrhenae Rhizoma 3.75g
山梔子 Gardeniae Fructus 3.75g
枸杞子 Lycii Fructus 3.75g
覆盆子 Rubi Fructus 3.75g
荊芥 Schizonepetae Spica 3.75g
防風 Saposhnikoviae Radix 3.75g
金銀花 Lonicerae Flos 3.75g

SY22 Rehmanniae Radix Preparata and Sophorae Radix Decoction
Sukjihwanggosam-tang 熟地黃苦蔘湯

Used to treat lower wasting-thirst.
• Retention of the placenta.

熟地黃 Rehmanniae Radix Preparata 15g
山茱萸 Corni Fructus 7.5g
白伏苓 Poria Sclerotium Alba 5.625g
澤瀉 Alismatis Rhizoma 5.625g
知母 Anemarrhenae Rhizoma 3.75g
黃栢 Phellodendri Cortex 3.75g
苦蔘 Sophorae Radix 3.75g

SY23 Akebiae Caulis Greatly Relieving Decoction
Moktongdaean-tang 木通大安湯

Used to treat puffy swelling.

木通 Akebiae Caulis 18.75g
生地黃 Rehmanniae Radix Crudus 18.75g
赤伏苓 Poria Sclerotium Rubra 7.5g
澤瀉 Alismatis Rhizoma 3.75g
車前子 Plantaginis Semen 3.75g
川黃連 Coptidis Rhizoma 3.75g
羌活 Osterici Radix 3.75g
防風 Saposhnikoviae Radix 3.75g
荊芥 Schizonepetae Spica 3.75g

SY24 Coptidis Rhizoma Intestine-Clearing Decoction
Hwangryeoncheongjang-tang 黃連淸腸湯

Used to treat dysentery.

生地黃 Rehmanniae Radix Crudus 15g
木通 Akebiae Caulis 7.5g
赤伏苓 Poria Sclerotium Rubra 7.5g
澤瀉 Alismatis Rhizoma 7.5g
猪苓 Polyporus 3.75g
車前子 Plantaginis Semen 3.75g
川黃連 Coptidis Rhizoma 3.75g
羌活 Osterici Radix 3.75g
防風 Saposhnikoviae Radix 3.75g

To treat strangury disease, remove 木通 Akebiae Caulis and add 3.75g of 荊芥 Schizonepetae Spica. It is called SY25 Hyeonggaecheongjang-tang 荊芥淸腸湯 Schizonepetae Spica Intestine- Cooling Decoction.

SY26 Cinnabaris Prime-Replenishing Powder
Jusaikwon-san 朱砂益元散

Used to flush summerheat.

滑石 Talcum 7.5g
澤瀉 Alismatis Rhizoma 3.75g
甘遂 Euphorbiae Kansui Radix 1.875g
朱砂 Cinnabaris 0.375g

Pulverize the above drugs. Take them with warm water.

SY27 Euphorbiae Kansui Radix Heaven-One Pill
Gamsucheonil-hwan 甘遂天一丸

Used to treat chest bind and immediate vomiting of ingested fluids

甘遂(末) Euphorbiae Kansui Radix (grind) 3.75g
輕粉(末) Calomelas (grind) 0.375g

Make ten pills with a flour paste and coat them with 朱砂 Cinnabaris. Pound them again when they are expected to take. Let the patient take them with water drawn from the well at daybreak. After three or four hours, if the patient does not have diarrhea, give two more pills. Diarrhea 3 times is desirable, and 5 or 6 times is better. Prepare a thin gruel, and after diarrhea, serve the gruel to the patient. If the preparation is not given, the patient will experience qi fall.

SY28

Calomelas and Euphorbiae Kansui Radix Dragon-Tiger Pellet

Gyeongbungamsuyongho-dan 輕粉甘遂龍虎丹

甘遂 Euphorbiae Kansui Radix 3.75g
輕粉 Calomelas 1.875g

Make ten pills.

SY29

Calomelas and Euphorbiae Kansui Radix Male-Female Pellet

Gyeongbungamsujawung-dan 輕粉甘遂雌雄丹

Used to flush summerheat.

輕粉 Calomelas equal amount
甘遂 Euphorbiae Kansui Radix equal amount

SY30

Olibanum, Myrrha, and Calomelas Pill

Yuhyangmolyakgyeongbun-hwan 乳香沒藥輕粉丸

輕粉 Calomelas 3.75g
乳香 Myrrha 1.875g
沒藥 Olibanum 1.875g
甘遂 Euphorbiae Kansui Radix 1.875g

Make thirty pills.
輕粉 Calomelas and 甘遂 Euphorbiae Kansui Radix are poisonous medicinals, so these cannot be taken much. 0.375g should be taken each time.

SY31

Calomelas, Olibanum, and Myrrha Pill

Gyeongbunyuhyangmolyak-hwan 輕粉乳香沒藥丸

輕粉 Calomelas 5.625g
乳香 Olibanum 1.875g
沒藥 Myrrha 1.875g
甘遂 Euphorbiae Kansui Radix 1.875g

SY32 White Tiger Decoction Baekho-tang 白虎湯

石膏 Gypsum Fibrosum 18.75g
知母 Anemarrhenae Rhizoma 7.5g
粳米 Oryzae Semen 90ml
甘草 Glycyrrhizae Radix et Rhizoma 2.625g

When 3.75g of 黃栢 Phellodendri Cortex is added, it is called SY33 Hwangbaekho- tang 黃白虎湯 Yellow-White Tiger Decoction.

SY34 Polyporus Decoction Jeoryeong-tang 猪苓湯

猪苓 Polyporus 3.75g
赤伏苓 Poria Sclerotium Rubra 3.75g
澤瀉 Alismatis Rhizoma 3.75g
滑石 Talcum 3.75g
阿膠 Asini Corii Colla 3.75g

SY35 Five Poria Powder Oryeong-san 五苓散

澤瀉 Alismatis Rhizoma 9.375g
赤伏苓 Poria Sclerotium Rubra 5.625g
猪苓 Polyporus 5.625g
白朮 Atractylodis Rhizoma Alba 5.625g
肉桂 Cinnamomi Cortex 1.875g

When 白朮 Atractylodis Rhizoma Alba and 肉桂 Cinnamomi Cortex are removed, it is called SY36 Saryeong-san 四令散 Four Poria Powder. This prescription appeared in Prescriptions of Zhang Zhongjing.

SY37 Kidney Qi Pill Singi-hwan 腎氣丸

It is a prescription that 五味子 Schisandrae Fructus is added to Yungmijihwang- tang 六味地黃湯 Six-flavor Rehmanniae Radix Preparata Decoction.

SY38 Coptidis Rhizoma and Pig Stomach Decoction
Hwangryeonjeodu-tang 黃連猪肚湯

雄猪肚 Male pig stomach 1 unit
黃連 Coptidis Rhizoma 187.5g
小麥 Tritici Semen 187.5g
天花粉 Trichosanthis Radix 187.5g
白伏神 Hoelen cum Pini Radix 150g

Pound the above medicines into powder and put them into the pig's stomach. Block the entry and put it into a steamer. After steaming, make them pills the size of the seed of an empress tree.

SY39 Diaphragm-Cooling Powder
Yanggyeok-san 凉隔散

Used to treat accumulated heat, agitation, mouth and tongue sores, red eyes, and clouded head.

連翹 Forsythiae Fructus 7.5g
大黃 Rhei Rhizoma 3.75g
芒硝 Natrii Sulfas 3.75g
薄荷 Menthae Herba 3.75g
甘草 Glycyrrhizae Radix et Rhizoma 3.75g
黃芩 Scutellariae Radix 3.75g

When 大黃 Rhei Rhizoma, 甘草 Glycyrrhizae Radix et Rhizoma, 黃芩 Scutellariae Radix is removed, it is called SY40 Leesiyanggyeok-san 李氏凉隔散 Lee's Diaphragm-Cooling Powder.

SY41 Six-Flavor Rehmanniae Radix Preparata Decoction
Yungmijihwang-tang 六味地黃湯

Used to treat consumptive disease.

熟地黃 Rehmanniae Radix Preparata 15g
枸杞子 Lycii Fructus 7.5g
山茱臾 Corni Fructus 7.5g
澤瀉 Alismatis Rhizoma 5.625g
牧丹皮 Moutan Cortex 5.625g
白伏苓 Poria Sclerotium Alba 5.625g

When 18.75g of glue of 民魚 Leiocassis Longirostris is added, it is called SY42 Hwaseokjihwang-tang 花惜地黃湯 Piteous Flower Rehmanniae Radix Preparata Decoction.

SY43 Rehmanniae Radix Crudus Decoction
Saengjihwang-tang 生地黃湯

Used to treat dim vision.

生地黃 Rehmanniae Radix Crudus 37.5g
熟地黃 Rehmanniae Radix Preparata 37.5g
玄蔘 Scrophulariae Radix 37.5g
石膏 Gypsum Fibrosum 37.5g

This prescription can be made a pasted pill as big as a seed of a paulownia. Take 50-70 pills with tea decoction on an empty stomach.

SY44 Lee's Red-Conducting Powder
Issidojeok-san 李氏導赤散

Used for urination that is like rice water. One is cured before taking it twice.

木通 Akebiae Caulis 3.75g
滑石 Talcum 3.75g
黃栢 Phellodendri Cortex 3.75g
赤伏苓 Poria Sclerotium Rubra 3.75g
生地黃 Rehmanniae Radix Crudus 3.75g
山梔子 Gardeniae Fructus 3.75g

SY45 Lee's Child-Plumping Pill
Issibia-hwan 李氏肥兒丸

Used to treat mild infantile malnutrition with accumulation.

胡黃連 Picrorhizae Rhizoma 18.75g
黃連 Coptidis Rhizoma 13.125g
神曲 Massa Medicata Fermentata 13.125g
麥芽 Hordei Fructus Germinatus 13.125g
白伏苓 Poria Sclerotium Alba 9.375g
蘆薈 Aloe 9.375g

Pulverize the above drugs. Make a pasted pill with Setariae Semen 黃米 as big as a mung bean. Take 20-30 pills with rice water.

SY46 Toxin-Dissolving Decoction Sodok-eum 消毒飮

Used to treat non-outthrust of seasonal pox, and resolve toxin.

牛蒡子 Arctii Fructus 7.5g
荊芥穗 Schizonepetae Flos 3.75g
防風 Saposhnikoviae Radix 1.875g

SY47 Hydrargyrum Nose-Fumigating Formula Sueunhunbi-bang 水銀薰鼻方

Used to treat red bayberry toxin sore, pemphigus, and throat-entwining wind.

黑鉛 Graphite 3.75g
水銀 Hydrargyrum 3.75g
朱砂 Cinnabaris 1.875g
乳香 Olibanum 1.875g
沒藥 Myrrha 1.875g
血竭 Draconis Sanguis 1.125g
石雄黃 Realgar 1.125g
硫黃 Sulfur 1.125g

Pulverize equal amounts of the drugs. Roll up into seven cigarette-like shapes. Make them seven. Place lamp burning scented oil on the table. The patient should lie in his bed with his whole body under a coverlet with his legs stretched. The patient has to hold cold water in his mouth and change it frequently in order to prevent damage to his mouth. Fumigate three times the first day and once a day from then on. After fumigating, the patient should not locate himself in cold area and be touched by wind. ○Sweating of vertex and cheek is desirable for throat-entwining wind.

SY48 Vermilionum Powder Yeongsa-san 靈砂散

Used to treat panting due to cold damage, chronic infantile convulsion, acute abdominal pain, and qi counterflow pattern.

靈砂 Vermilionum 0.375 or 0.5625g

Take this drug with warm water.

SY49 Pufferfish Roe Powder Donlan-san 豚卵散

Used to treat brain flat-abscess, head sore.

河豚卵 Pufferfish Roe

Pulverize the above drug.

SY50 Eye Drop Powder Jeoman-san 點眼散

黃連 Coptidis Rhizoma

Mix this medicine with human milk. Steam and extract juice from it. Drop the juice in the eyes or take it.

SY51 Delivery-Inducing Powder Cheosaeng-san 催生散

Used to treat difficult delivery.
- Bleeding of gum and nose. In emergency circumstances, heat this medicine and apply to heels.

香油 Elsholtziae Herba

SY52 Major Euphorbiae Kansui Radix Powder Daegamsu-san 大甘遂散

Used to treat major chest bind.

甘遂末 Euphorbiae Kansui Radix (grind) 1.875g

When the weight of 甘遂 Euphorbiae Kansui Radix decreases to 1.125g, it is called SY53 Sogamsu-san 小甘遂散 Euphorbiae Kansui Radix Minor Powder.
This prescription is used to treat minor chest bind.

SY54 Kidney-Restoring Speech-Releasing Decoction Guisinhaeeo-tang 歸腎解語湯

Used to treat wind stroke with loss of speech.

荆芥 Schizonepetae Spica equal amount
防風 Saposhnikoviae Radix equal amount
羌活 Osterici Radix equal amount
獨活 Angelicae Continentalis Radix equal amount
薄荷 Menthae Herba a quantity

• Decoct the medicines with water and put them under a table to fumigate for nose. The patient will be able to speak after some time.

SY55 New Bupleuri Radix Minor Decoction Sinsosiho-tang 新小柴胡湯

Used to treat overexertion after sexual activity or sexual activity after overexertion, greater yang exterior pattern, and lesser yang initial pattern.

熟地黃 Rehmanniae Radix Preparata 11.25g
柴胡 Bupleuri Radix 7.5g
前胡 Angelicae Decusivae Radix 3.75g
玄蔘 Scrophulariae Radix 3.75g
白伏苓 Poria Sclerotium Alba 3.75g

• Or 知母 Anemarrhenae Rhizoma can be replaced 白伏苓 Poria Sclerotium Alba.

SY56 New Bupleuri Radix Major Decoction Sindaesiho-tang 新大柴胡湯

Used to treat lesser yang cramp, yang brightness constipation, delirious speech, tidal fever, and absence of sweating.

柴胡 Bupleuri Radix 15g
前胡 Angelicae Decursivae Radix 9.375g
知母 Anemarrhenae Rhizoma 9.375g
芒硝 Natrii Sulfas 5.625g
防風 Saposhnikoviae Radix 5.625g

SY57 Scrophulariae Radix White Tiger Decoction Hyeonsambaekho-tang 玄蔘白虎湯

Used to treat yin collapse; delirious speech, fecal block, and stirring wind. If the symptoms are acute, 9.375g of 靈芝 Ganoderma and 9.375g of 芒硝 Natrii Sulfas can be added.

熟地黃 Rehmanniae Radix Preparata 37.5 or 56.25g
石膏 Gypsum Fibrosum 22.5 or 37.5g
玄蔘 Scrophulariae Radix 15g
生地黃 Rehmanniae Radix Crudus 15g
柴胡 Bupleuri Radix 9.375g
知母 Anemarrhenae Rhizoma 9.375g
山茱萸 Corni Fructus 5.625g
防風 Saposhnikoviae Radix 5.625g
覆盆子 Rubi Fructus 5.625g
獨活 Angelicae Continentalis Radix 5.625g

SY58 Yin-Lowering White Tiger Decoction Gangeumbaekho-tang 降陰白虎湯

Used to treat yin collapse, delirious speech, fecal block, and wind about to stir.

熟地黃 Rehmanniae Radix Preparata 22.5 or 37.5g
石膏 Gypsum Fibrosum 22.5 or 37.5g
柴胡 Bupleuri Radix 15g
前胡 Angelicae Decursivae Radix 15g
生地黃 Rehmaniae Radix Crudus 15g
知母 Anemarrhenae Rhizoma 9.375g
玄蔘 Scrophulariae Radix 9.375g
防風 Saposhnikoviae Radix 9.375g
獨活 Angelicae Continentalis Radix 5.625g
芒硝 Natrii Sulfas 5.625g

SY59 Exterior Symtoms White Tiger Decoction Pyojeungbaekho-tang 表症白虎湯

This prescription is that 15g of 柴胡 Bupleuri Radix is added to SY18 Jihwangbaekho-tang 地黃白虎湯 Rehmanniae Radix Crudus White Tiger Decoction.

SY60 Rehmanniae Radix Black Turtoise Decoction Jihwanghyeonmu-tang 地黃玄武湯

Used to treat acute patterns of yin collapse, fever, diarrhea, delirious speech, and agitation.

熟地黃 Rehmanniae Radix Preparata 37.5g
石膏 Gypsum Fibrosum 22.5 or 37.5g
赤伏苓 Poria Sclerotium Rubra 7.5g
生地黃 Rehmanniae Radix Crudus 7.5g
柴胡 Bupleuri Radix 7.5g
山茱萸 Corni Fructus 7.5g
知母 Anemarrhenae Rhizoma 7.5g
防風 Saposhnikoviae Radix 5.625g
黃連 Coptidis Rhizoma 5.625g
澤瀉 Alismatis Rhizoma 5.625g
覆盆子 Rubi Fructus 5.625g
獨活 Angelicae Continentalis Radix 5.625g

SY61 Lactation-Inducing Kidney-Restoring Decoction Tongyuguisin-tang 通乳歸腎湯

猪蹄 Pettitoes 4 pairs
通草 Tetrapanacis Medulla 3.75g
荊芥 Schizonepetae Spica 3.75g
熟地黃 Rehmanniae Radix Preparata 3.75g
防風 Saposhnikoviae Radix 3.75g

Decoct without residue. Take this prescription as required to promote lactation.

SY62 Fetus-Protecting Rehmanniae Radix Preparata Decoction Botaejihwang-tang 保胎地黃湯

Used to treat fetal spotting and bleeding.

民魚膠 glue of Leiocassis Longirostris 18.75g
熟地黃 Rehmanniae Radix Preparata 15g
山藥 Dioscoreae Rhizoma 7.5g
山茱萸 Corni Fructus 7.5g
澤瀉 Alismatis Rhizoma 5.625g
牧丹皮 Moutan Cortex 5.625g
白伏苓 Poria Sclerotium (white) 5.625g
糯米 Oryzae Semen 20g

Empirical Prescriptions for Soyang Type 少陰人 經驗方

SY-e1 Scrophulariae Radix Toxin-Repelling Powder Hyeonsampaedok-san 玄蔘敗毒散

Used to treat fever, aversion to cold, headache, generalized pain, and agitation.

- Initial and second pain of cold damage, interior heat, ascending counterflow, and vomiting.

羌活 Osterici Radix 5.625g
獨活 Angelicae Continentalis Radix 5.625g
荊芥 Schizonepetae Spica 5.625g
防風 Saposhnikoviae Radix 5.625g
柴胡 Bupleuri Radix 5.625g
玄蔘 Scrophulariae Radix 5.625g
前胡 Angelicae Decursivae Radix 5.625g
梔子 Gardeniae Fructus 5.625g
薄荷 Menthae Herba 5.625g
忍冬藤 Lonicerae Folium et Caulis 3.75g
地骨皮 Lycii Cortex 3.75g

SY-e2 Saposhnikoviae Radix Unblocking Holy Powder Bangpungtongseong-san 防風通聖散

Used to treat interior heat, yin deficiency stirring fire; wasting-thirst, and disease of face, eye, mouth, nose, and tooth.

- Mild infantile malnutrition, fat and thin.

滑石 Talcum 1.875g
生地黃 Rehmanniae Radix Crudus 1.875g
防風 Saposhnikoviae Radix 1.875g
石膏 Gypsum Fibrosum 1.875g
羌活 Osterici Radix 1.875g
獨活 Angelicae Continentalis Radix 1.875g
柴胡 Bupleuri Radix 1.875g
前胡 Angelicae Decursivae Radix 1.875g
薄荷 Menthae Herba 1.875g
荊芥 Schizonepetae Spica 1.875g
惡實 Arctii Fructus 1.875g
山梔子 Gardeniae Fructus 1.875g

SY-e3 Thousand Gold Pieces Red-Conducting Powder
Cheongeumdojeok-san 千金導赤散

Used to treat exterior pattern, alternating chills and fever, inability to urinate or defecate for one day.

生地黃 Rehmanniae Radix Crudus 15g
木通 Akebiae Caulis 7.5g
黃連 Coptidis Rhizoma 7.5g
柴胡 Bupleuri Radix 7.5g
山梔子 Gardeniae Fructus 7.5g
覆盆子 Rubi Fructus 7.5g

SY-e4 Bupleuri Radix and Trichosanthis Semen Decoction
Sihogwaru-tang 柴胡栝蔞湯

Used to treat alternating chills and fever, sweating, shortness of breath, delirious speech, chest bind, dry throat, dizzy vision, and deafness.

生地黃 Rehmanniae Radix Crudus 15g
木通 Akebiae Caulis 3.75g
栝蔞仁 Trichosanthis Semen 3.75g
山茱萸 Corni Fructus 3.75g
覆盆子 Rubi Fructus 3.75g
黃連 Coptidis Rhizoma 3.75g
苦蔘 Sophorae Radix 3.75g
柴胡 Bupleuri Radix 3.75g
前胡 Angelicae Decursivae Radix 3.75g
獨活 Angelicae Continentalis Radix 3.75g

SY-e5 Bupleuri Radix Four Poria Decoction
Sihosaryeong-tang 柴胡四苓湯

Used to treat abdominal pain due to cold damage.
• Abdominal pain, summerheat diarrhea or constipation for three days.

柴胡 Bupleuri Radix 7.5g
澤瀉 Alismatis Rhizoma 7.5g
猪苓 Polyporus 7.5g
赤伏苓 Poria Sclerotium (red) 7.5g
黃連 Coptidis Rhizoma 3.75g
栝蔞仁 Trichosanthis Semen 3.75g
滑石 Talcum 3.75g
車前子 Plantaginis Semen 3.75g

SY-e6 Simple White Tiger Decoction Danbaekho-tang 單白虎湯

Used to treat more fever than cold, constipation, deep multiple abscess, throat disease due to yang toxin, yellow flat-abscess, and disease of face, eye, mouth, nose, and tooth.

石膏 Gypsum Fibrosum 15g
生地黃 Rehmanniae Radix Crudus 15g
知母 Anemarrhenae Rhizoma 7.5g

SY-e7 Sea-Wading White Tiger Decoction Dohaebaekho-tang 渡海白虎湯

Used to treat three yang patter, grimy facial complexion, headache, delirious speech, more heat, vexation in the chest, and fecal block.

石膏 Gypsum Fibrosum 15g
生地黃 Rehmanniae Radix Crudus 7.5g
知母 Anemarrhenae Rhizoma 7.5g
覆盆子 Rubi Fructus 7.5g
山茱萸 Corni Fructus 7.5g
肉從蓉 Cistnachis Herba 7.5g
苦蔘 Sophorae Radix 3.75g
枸杞子 Lycii Fructus 3.75g

SY-e8 Embellished Brocade White Tiger Decoction Geumsangcheomhwabaekho-tang 錦上添花白虎湯

This medicine has the same usage as SY-e7 Dohaebaekho-tang 渡海白虎湯 Sea-Wading White Tiger Decoction.

石膏 Gypsum Fibrosum 15g
生地黃 Rehmanniae Radix Crudus 15g
知母 Anemarrhenae Rhizoma 3.75g
山茱萸 Corni Fructus 3.75g
覆盆子 Rubi Fructus 3.75g

SY-e9 Polyporus White Tiger Decoction Jeoryeongbaekho-tang 猪苓白虎湯

This medicine has the same usage as SY6 Jeryeongchajeonja-tang 猪苓車前子湯 Polyporus and Plantaginis Semen Decoction.

石膏 Gypsum Fibrosum 15g
生地黃 Rehmanniae Radix Crudus 15g
知母 Anemarrhenae Rhizoma 11.25g
黃栢 Phellodendri Cortex 3.75g
澤瀉 Alismatis Rhizoma 3.75g
猪苓 Polyporus 3.75g
赤伏苓 Poria Sclerotium 3.75g

SY-e10 Eight-Flavor Sophorae Radix Decoction Palmigosam-tang 八味苦蔘湯

Used to treat cold damage, abdominal pain excluding diarrhea or constipation for three days after defecation.

- Abdominal pain, stuffiness and fullness, hematemesis, vomiting, and interior pattern.
- This prescription should be used in yin pattern.

生地黃 Rehmanniae Radix Crudus 15g
苦蔘 Sophorae Radix 3.75g
知母 Anemarrhenae Rhizoma 3.75g
山茱萸 Corni Fructus 3.75g
覆盆子 Rubi Fructus 3.75g
赤伏苓 Poria Sclerotium 3.75g
澤瀉 Alismatis Rhizoma 3.75g
牧丹皮 Moutan Cortex 3.75g

SY-e11 Seven-Flavor Polyporus Decoction Chilmijeoryung-tang 七味猪苓湯

Used to treat yin deficiency stirring fire, afternoon tidal fever and steaming bone.

生地黃 Rehmanniae Radix Crudus 15g
山茱萸 Corni Fructus 7.5g
覆盆子 Rubi Fructus 7.5g
澤瀉 Alismatis Rhizoma 7.5g
赤伏苓 Poria Sclerotium 7.5g
猪苓 Polyporus 3.75g
黃栢 Phellodendri Cortex 3.75g

- To treat abdominal pain, stuffiness and fullness, and vomiting, add 3.75g of 牧丹皮 Moutan Cortex. It is called SY-e12 Palmijeoryung-tang 八味猪苓湯 Eight-Flavor Polyporus Decoction.

SY-e13

Water-Fire Forded Decoction

Suhwagije-tang 水火既濟湯

Used to treat yin deficiency stirring fire, afternoon tidal fever, and initial transmutational symptoms like wasting-thirst syndrome, welling-abscess and flat-abscess of face, eye, mouth, nose and tooth.

- For the infant presenting polyphagia but emaciation, doctors should ask whether there is mild bleeding between two teeth before using this prescription.

生地黃 Rehmanniae Radix Crudus 3.75g
乾地黃 Rehmanniae Radix Siccus 3.75g
知母 Anemarrhenae Rhizoma 3.75g
黃栢 Phellodendri Cortex 3.75g
山茱萸 Corni Fructus 3.75g
覆盆子 Rubi Fructus 3.75g
柴胡 Bupleuri Radix 3.75g
苦蔘 Sophorae Radix 3.75g
伏苓 Poria Sclerotium 3.75g
澤瀉 Alismatis Rhizoma 3.75g
肉蓯蓉 Cistanchis Herba 3.75g

SY-e14

Cooling-Chilling Fire-Dissipating Decoction

Cheongryangsanhwa-tang 淸凉散火湯

忍冬 Lonicerae Folium 15g
苦蔘 Sophorae Radix 7.5g
生地黃 Rehmanniae Radix Crudus 3.75g
覆盆子 Rubi Fructus 3.75g
薄荷 Menthae Herba 3.75g
山梔子 Gardeniae Fructus 3.75g
防風 Saposhnikoviae Radix 3.75g
石膏 Gypsum Fibrosum 3.75g
荊芥 Schizonepetae Spica 1.875g
牛蒡子 Arctii Fructus 1.875g

SY-e15

Akebiae Caulis and Sophorae Radix Decoction

Moktonggosam-tang 木通苦蔘湯

Used to treat puffy swelling and tympanites. If this medicine is ineffectual, it is a incurable disease.

木通 Akebiae Caulis 22.5g
生地黃 Rehmanniae Radix Crudus 15g
苦蔘 Sophorae Radix 3.75g
黃栢 Phellodendri Cortex 3.75g
車前子 Plantaginis Semen 3.75g

SY-e16 Bupleuri Radix Abdomden-Cooling Decoction Sihocheongbok-tang 柴胡淸腹湯

Used to treat dysentery.

黃連 Coptidis Rhizoma 11.25g
生地黃 Rehmanniae Radix Crudus 11.25g
木通 Akebiae Caulis 7.5g
羌活 Osterici Radix 3.75g
柴胡 Bupleuri Radix 3.75g
澤瀉 Alismatis Rhizoma 3.75g
猪苓 Polyporus 3.75g
赤伏苓 Poria Sclerotium 3.75g

SY-e17 White Tiger Decoction Paste Baekhotang-go 白虎湯膏

Used to treat toxin swelling, and wind pattern.

石膏 Gypsum Fibrosum equal amount
生地黃 Rehmanniae Radix Crudus equal amount
知母 Anemarrhenae Rhizoma equal amount
澤瀉 Alismatis Rhizoma equal amount

- Stew and remove the dregs. Make the decoction into paste. Add 輕粉 Calomelas, 乳香 Olibanum, and 沒藥 Myrrha. And make them into pasted pills.

SY-e18 White Tiger Prime-Replenishing Powder Baekhoikwon-san 白虎益元散

Used to treat summerheat syndrome.

滑石 Talcum 9.375g
白虎膏 White tiger paste 3.75g
朱砂 Cinnabaris 3.75g

SY-e19 Soyang Stomach-Tonifying Decoction
Soyangbowi-tang 少陽補胃湯

Used to treat counterflow qi, abdominal pain, and headache.

熟地黃 Rehmanniae Radix Preparata 15g
山茱萸 Corni Fructus 5.625g
赤伏苓 Poria Sclerotium 5.625g
澤瀉 Alismatis Rhizoma 5.625g
車前子 Plantaginis Semen 3.75g
知母 Anemarrhenae Rhizoma 3.75g
羌活 Osterici Radix 3.75g
獨活 Angelicae Continentalis Radix 3.75g
荊芥 Schizonepetae Spica 3.75g
防風 Saposhnikoviae Radix 3.75g

SY-e20 Rehmanniae Radix Crudus Toxin-Repelling Powdera
Jihwangpaedok-san 地黃敗毒散

Used to treat interior pattern; panting.
• Yang brightness, triple yang combination disease.

生地黃 Rehmanniae Radix Crudus 15g
知母 Anemarrhenae Rhizoma 7.5g
赤伏苓 Poria Sclerotium 3.75g
澤瀉 Alismatis Rhizoma 3.75g
猪苓 Polyporus 3.75g
滑石 Talcum 3.75g
車前子 Plantaginis Semen 3.75g
羌活 Osterici Radix 3.75g
獨活 Angelicae Continentalis Radix 3.75g
防風 Saposhnikoviae Radix 3.75g
荊芥 Schizonepetae Spica 3.75g
苽蔞仁 Trichosanthis Semen 3.75g

SY-e21 Rehmanniae Radix Crudus Decoction
Jihwang-tang 地黃湯

Used to treat swellings and sores.

生地黃 Rehmanniae Radix Crudus 7.5g
木通 Akebiae Caulis 7.5g
滑石 Talcum 3.75g
赤伏苓 Poria Sclerotium 3.75g
山梔子 Gardeniae Fructus 3.75g
牛蒡子 Arctii Fructus 3.75g
荊芥 Schizonepetae Spica 3.75g
防風 Saposhnikoviae Radix 3.75g

When 11.25g of 忍冬藤 Lonicerae Folium et Caulis, 7.5g of 連翹 Forsythiae Fructus, 3.75g of 苦蔘 Sophorae Radix, 3.75g of 石膏 Gypsum Fibrosum, 3.75g of 金銀花 Lonicerae Flos, 3.75g of 薄荷 Menthae Herba, 3.75g of 地骨皮 Lycii Cortex, and 1.875g of 柴胡 Bupleuri Radix are added, the efficiency of the medicine will get better.

SY-e22 Transformation-Helping Pellet Chanhwa-dan 贊化丹

Used to treat pestilence, mental derangement, aggregation-accumulation, fright epilepsy, malaria, puffy swelling, dysuria, headache, abdominal pain, food stagnation, stuffiness and fullness, diarrhea, jaundice, and infantile malnutrition. It can be used to treat widespread symptoms except pregnant women. It can be taken for malign sores. To treat constipation, take this medicine with a decoction of 芒硝 Natrii Sulfas.

熟地黃 Rehmanniae Radix Preparata 93.75g
山茱萸 Corni Fructus 11.25g
牧丹皮 Moutan Cortex 11.25g
澤瀉 Alismatis Rhizoma 11.25g
蘆薈(煆) Aloe (calcine) 11.25g
木通 Akebiae Caulis 11.25g
苦蔘 Sophorae Radix 11.25g
玄蔘 Scrophulariae Radix 11.25g
柴胡 Bupleuri Radix 11.25g
前胡 Angelicae Decursivae Radix 11.25g
荊芥 Schizonepetae Spica 11.25g
防風 Saposhnikoviae Radix 11.25g
連翹 Forsythiae Fructus 11.25g
牛蒡子 Arctii Fructus 11.25g
紫菀 Asteris Radix 11.25g
黃連 Coptidis Rhizoma 11.25g
神曲 Massa Medicata Fermentata 11.25g
麥芽 Hordei Fructus Germinatus 11.25g
忍冬藤 Lonicerae Folium et Caulis 11.25g
栝蔞仁 Trichosanthis Semen 11.25g
甘遂 Euphorbiae Kansui Radix 11.25g

First, put 熟地黃 Rehmanniae Radix Preparata into water of 薄荷 Menthae Herba and decoct it to make paste. Then pound the rest medicines 1000 times in a mortar. Make 40 pills from the resulting mixture and coat them with 朱砂 Cinnabaris. 5-9 pills should be taken with spring water or warm water.

SY-e23 Rehmanniae Radix Preparata Added Decoction Gamijihwang-tang 加味地黃湯

Used to treat menstrual irregularities and black colored menstrual flow.
- To treat constipation, add 37.5g of 石膏 Gypsum Fibrosum.
- To treat dysuria, add 18.75g of 澤瀉 Alismatis Rhizoma.

熟地黃 Rehmanniae Radix Preparata 15g
生地黃 Rehmanniae Radix Crudus 15g
山茱萸 Corni Fructus 7.5g
白伏苓 Poria Sclerotium (white) 7.5g
澤瀉 Alismatis Rhizoma 7.5g
牧丹皮 Moutan Cortex 7.5g
玄蔘 Scrophulariae Radix 7.5g
羌活 Osterici Radix 3.75g
獨活 Angelicae Continentalis Radix 3.75g
荊芥 Schizonepetae Spica 3.75g
防風 Saposhnikoviae Radix 3.75g

SY-e24 Fire-Dissipating Added Decoction Gamisanhwa-tang 加味散火湯

Used to treat disease of the throat.

- To treat stagnation and disturbing influence, add 11.25g of 苦蔘 Sophorae Radix.
- To treat eye disease, add 7.5g of 黃栢 Phellodendri Cortex.
- To treat abdominal pain caused by accumulation, add 11.25g of 苦蔘 Sophorae Radix.

石膏 Gypsum Fibrosum 18.75g
生地黃 Rehmanniae Radix Crudus 7.5g
忍冬藤 Lonicerae Folium et Caulis 7.5g
連翹 Forsythiae Fructus 7.5g
山梔子 Gardeniae Fructus 3.75g
薄荷 Menthae Herba 3.75g
知母 Anemarrhenae Rhizoma 3.75g
防風 Saposhnikoviae Radix 3.75g
荊芥 Schizonepetae Spica 3.75g

SY-e25 White Tiger Added Decoction Gamibaekho-tang 加味白虎湯

Used to treat headache continued for a long time, constipation.

- To treat diarrhea, add 7.5g of 澤瀉 Alismatis Rhizoma. This prescription also can be used to treat heat pain of the penis.

石膏 Gypsum Fibrosum 37.5g
生地黃 Rehmanniae Radix Crudus 15g
知母 Anemarrhenae Rhizoma 11.25g
黃栢 Phellodendri Cortex 7.5g
荊芥 Schizonepetae Spica 3.75g
防風 Saposhnikoviae Radix 3.75g

SY-e26 Dual Principle Decoction Yangui-jeon 兩儀煎

Used to treat cold and impediment of the penis.

熟地黃 Rehmanniae Radix Preparata 75g
山茱萸 Corni Fructus 37.5g

SY-e27 Menthae Herba Decoction Bakha-jeon 薄荷煎

Used to treat stagnant qi.

薄荷 Menthae Herba 11.25g
苦蔘 Sophorae Radix 7.5g

SY-e28 Rehmanniae Radix Preparata Added Decoction[12] Gamijihwang-tang 加味地黃湯

Used to treat impotence and ascending counterflow pattern.

熟地黃 Rehmanniae Radix Preparata 11.25g
山茱萸 Corni Fructus 11.25g
白伏苓 Poria Sclerotium (white) 7.5g
車前子 Plantaginis Semen 7.5g
澤瀉 Alismatis Rhizoma 7.5g
兎絲子 Cuscutae Semen 7.5g
羌活 Osterici Radix 3.75g
獨活 Angelicae Continentalis Radix 3.75g
玄蔘 Scrophulariae Radix 3.75g
忍冬藤 Lonicerae Folium et Caulis 3.75g
薄荷 Menthae Herba 3.75g

12) This prescription has different ingredients with SY-e23 Gamijihwang-tang.

Daily Health Maintenance using Sasang Constitutional Theory

Everyone should have been able to roughly identify their own constitution after reading the previous chapter. Let us now think about how we can apply the information.

In each constitution, there are certain emotions that warrant caution and certain principles to regulate these emotions. There are certain foods that are to be avoided and foods that are appropriate. There are herbs that are either beneficial or harmful to one's constitution, and there are certain principles to treat diseases as well as rules for longevity that allow a person to acquire lifelong health.

Knowing one's constitution is not only helpful for physical health but also for harmonious social and family life. This is because each constitution has different characteristics which allow one to recognize his abilities and temperament as well as the merits and demerits of one's personality. Through such means, one can regulate one's mind and behavior, and thus maintain a healthy mind and body. Additionally, by knowing which things to be aware of, a person can confidently deal with everyday affairs. One's understanding of others will also deepen so that one can develop the good habit of giving warm consideration to others, leading to better overall relationships.

Clearly there are many things to be gained through understanding constitutions. In this chapter, I will be presenting a few health cultivation methods that can be easily applied to one's daily life.

1. Beneficial and Harmful Foods

Traditionally it is said that food and medicine have the same origin. This implies that diet is just as important as medicine in the treatment and prevention of disease.

As foods have less of an energetic variance than medicine, it can be said that they act more mildly on the body. It is clear, however, that there are beneficial and harmful foods according to each constitution. Nevertheless, since foods are taken for a long period of time, they are even more important than medicine. Foods that are appropriate for the constitution are the best tonic, but those that are inappropriate will become toxins that gradually accumulate in the body and cause disease.

Eating foods that are appropriate for the constitution will suppress the strength of organs that have excessive energy and will strengthen organs that are deficient. This will result in harmonious balance. Yang types will be induced to Yin tendencies and Yin types will be induced to Yang tendencies so that both types can achieve balance.

What vegetables make the best morning juice? What kind of fruits will be good to us? What tonics are the best? Is there any food that is especially harmful? Are there certain guidelines to follow as a fundamental principle in selecting proper foods? These are questions that people frequently ask.

Some foods supply energy while others have a medicinal effect. Both of these actions are taken into consideration in SCM. This encourages us to be scrupulous in the selection of daily foods and to better understand those foods that supplement our constitutional weaknesses or imbalances.

This does not mean that you cannot have foods that are not appropriate for your constitution. It only means that you should eat more foods that are appropriate for your constitution. For instance, if you want to add a special health food to your diet, it should be selected from the foods recognized by SCM to benefit your particular constitution. Your diet should also be regulated if you habitually over eat foods inappropriate for your constitution.

Many people in their middle and older years attempt to supplement their diets with vegetable juices or mixtures of eggs, apples and oranges. They do this because they feel that there is something lacking in their diet. They believe that their health will improve if they change or supplement their usual diet. The real question is, however, what determines the standard by which proper foods are selected

One example is that many people eat chicken because it is known to have high nutritional value. In Korea, chicken soup made with ginseng is popular as a summertime nutritional boost. Unfortunately, the SY-type persons need to avoid this kind of soup because, in severe cases they can develop skin rashes and red eyes. Even if a SY-type person does not have these adverse reactions, he or she is still recommended not to eat chicken or take ginseng as a tonic for an extended period of time. Western medicine would attribute these symptoms to allergic reactions, but SCM systematically explains the method of selecting the correct foods for each constitution.

Western medicine uses diet therapy as well. Patients with abnormal liver functions, for example, are advised to eat foods that are high in protein and low in fat. They are advised to ingest large amounts of fish, including shellfish. Thus, the dietary measures in western medicine vary depending on a patient's condition. SCM uses the diet in a different way. It does not deal with specific diseases per se, instead it discusses the proper method to regulating and balancing one's constitution.

In general, cold foods and drinks are not appropriate for Yin types and warm foods and drinks are not appropriate for Yang types. People who develop abdominal pain and/or diarrhea after ingesting many cold summer fruits, like watermelon or muskmelon, or cold drinks, like draft beers or soft drinks, are generally of the SE constitutional type. Since they have weak digestive systems and cold bodies, foods that are cold or hard to digest are not good for them. On the contrary, foods that are easy to digest or warm, like chicken, are appropriate for them and can warm up their cold bodies.

When preparing foods, the SE-type persons are advised to use stimulating condiments to help increase the appetite and digestion and to avoid using large amounts of oil or eating bland food. SE-type persons should develop a habit of enjoying warm drinks or foods. Even in summer, it is better to drink warm water than to drink ice cold water.

The SY-type persons have a good digestive system, so they digest all kinds of food easily. Even in winter, they have no troubles with cold foods like cold buckwheat noodles or cold drinks. Parents of SY-type children do not need to worry even if their child enjoys eating ice cream in the winter. Though there may be a concern for tooth decay, it is rare that the SY-type persons develop digestive problems from eating ice cream.

SY-type persons do not usually have trouble selecting foods. They are not fussy eaters and have a good appetite and good digestion. But since they have a great deal of heat in their constitution, they must carefully avoid foods that induce heat in the body. Foods that are appropriate for the SE-type persons, such as chicken and honey, are actually harmful for SY-type persons.

Since the question of digestion is not a concern for the SY-type persons, they should select foods based on their temperature. Because the SY-type persons easily develop a deficiency of Yin, foods that have the ability to nourish Yin are recommended. In terms of grains and legumes, barley, aduki beans and mung beans are best for them.

Like the the SY type, TY-type persons are also advised to ingest fresh, cold foods. The difference is that the SY-type persons have a vigorous digestive function that can handle fatty foods, whereas the

TY-type persons are better suited with plain foods. Foods that are low in fat and bland foods without added spices are appropriate for the TY type.

Since the TY-type persons have a weak liver function, if they regularly ingest foods high in calories and high in protein, which can overburden the liver, they can develop liver problems.

The TE-type persons have a weak Upper Burner and so are susceptible to respiratory and circulatory system disorders. They are usually overweight and thus should avoid foods that are known to cause heart disease or stroke. Also they are encouraged to ingest foods which can strengthen their weak lung function.

For them, foods that are rich in protein are recommended in stead of fatty foods. But as they have the habit of overeating, the TE-type persons are susceptible to obesity, hypertension and constipation. Thus they must avoid foods that are stimulating and fatty. Moreover, they should avoid over eating even the foods appropriate to their constitution and exercise regularly or take saunas to promote sweating and prevent obesity. It is also important for the TE-type person to keep proper dietary measures to eliminate habitual constipation.

The following is a list of grains, meats, seafood, vegetables and fruits that are appropriate for each constitution:

① The Taeyang (TY) type

For the TY-type persons, foods that are plain or bland or foods that strengthen the liver and nourish Yin are appropriate. Seafood and vegetables, which are low in fat, are especially good.

· Grains: buckwheat
· Seafood: shrimp, oyster, abalone, wreath shell, crab, sea cucumber, crucian carp
· Vegetables: watershield plant, pine needles
· Fruits: grapes, wild grapes, actinidia fruit, persimmons, cherries,

Chinese quince, pine pollen

* Harmful Foods: those that are pungent and hot or greasy

② The Soyang (SY) type

Since the SY-type persons have a lot of heat in their bodies, seafood, vegetables and foods that are fresh and cold are beneficial. Since their bodies can easily develop Yin deficiency, foods that nourish Yin are good.

· Grains/legumes: barley, aduki beans, mung beans
· Meat/poultry: pork, eggs, duck
· Seafood: oyster, sea cucumber, sea squirt, abalone, shrimp, crab, swellfish, lobster, carp, snakeheaded fish (mullet), tortoise, flatfish,
· Vegetables: Chinese cabbage, cucumber, lettuce, burdock, pumpkin, eggplant, carrots
· Fruits: watermelon, musk melon, strawberries, bananas, pineapple
· Others: beer, iced drinks

* Harmful foods: pungent, stimulating condiments such as hot pepper, ginger, green onion, garlic, mustard, curry, etc. chicken, goat meat, honey, ginseng

③ The Taeeum (TE) type

The TE-type persons generally have large bodies and a good digestive system. Thus they are recommended to ingest foods that are high in either animal or vegetable protein.

· Grains/legumes: wheat, beans, yams, Job's tear, millet, peanuts, perilla seeds, sugar,
· brown rice
· Meat/poultry: beef, milk, butter, cheese
· Seafood: cod liver oil, spawn of pollack, mud snail, eel, cod, brown seaweed, kelp, laver
· Fruits/nuts: chestnuts, pine nuts, walnuts, gingko nuts, pear, ume

plum, apricot, plum
· Vegetables: radishes, broad bellflower, carrots, glehnia root, braken, lotus roots, taro, yams, mushrooms

* Harmful foods: chicken, pork, ginseng, honey, ginger

④ The Soeum (SE) type

Since the SE-type persons can easily develop stomach disturbances due to a weak digestive system, spices and warm foods are good for them. Fatty foods, cold foods and raw foods can easily cause diarrhea.

· Grains: glutinous rice, glutinous millet, potatoes
· Fruits: apples, oranges, tomatoes, peaches, dates
· Meat/poultry: chicken, deer meat, sparrow, pheasant, goat's milk, goat, lamb, honey
· Seafood: Alaskan Pollack, red snapper, anchovy, croaker, mud snail
· Vegetables: spinach, cabbage, dropwort, green onion, garlic, ginger, red pepper, mustard, black pepper, curry

* Harmful foods: cold noodles, musk melon, watermelon, cold milk, ice cream, beer, barley, pork, cuttlefish, wheat products

2. Preserving health by exercising adequate mental control

The ancient physicians recognized that diseases were caused by digestive pathologies due to intemperate ingestion of food or contraction of external pathogenic Qi (namely Wind, Cold, Summerheat, Dampness, Dryness, Fire, Heat, etc.), but they overlooked the effect of the mind on the body, how love, hatred, desires, joy, anger, sorrow, and pleasure could induce deviations and cause illness.

The Sasang constitutional medicine (SCM) does not deny that

external factors contribute to pathogenesis. However, even among those living in the same environment and eating the same food, some manage to stay healthy while some become sick. In light of the fact that different people are affected differently by the same conditions, it would be inaccurate to believe that the external factors are the sole determinants involved in pathologic development. For instance, those who were born with a "cold" and "weak" digestive system could experience indigestion after ingesting cold foods, while those who have a constitutionally "strong" digestive system can remain fine after taking the same food.

In the Sasang medicine point of view, the "weak digestive system" or the "weak circulatory/respiratory system" are not merely related to only the physical organs of an individual. It emphasizes the intricate association between the organs of the Four Affiliations (Lung, Spleen, Liver, and Kidney) and the emotional deviations (Sorrow, Anger, Joy, and Pleasure). The structural scheme and balance of the Four Organ Systems are affected by the variations and deviations of the Four Emotions, and vice versa.

Naturally, it is equally important to control the *Seong-Jeong*, or the dichotomous mental deviations, in addition to controlling the energy of the physical organs in order to treat the diseases of the body. In the same context as the famous SCM saying, "Control the mind, and so control the disease (治心治病)", the first step in preventing and curing illness would be to control one's own *Seong-Jeong*.

The Taeyang (TY) constitutional type persons tend to respond easily to belittlement or scorn with anger. It may be helpful to learn to breathe in and out and calm down as they feel the rush of anger flare up, until the angry moment passes away and dwindles down. It they can train themselves to do this every time and restrain from bursting out over trivialities, they could remain unscathed from the ravages of the flame of anger on the physical body.

They can be very bold and enterprising, prone to underestimate the setbacks involved in a task. It must be remembered that it is important to preexamine and premeditate, planning it out carefully before entering into the challenge. Also, it should be understood that nothing can be rushed, especially if the task spans beyond one's capacity or qualifications. Though charismatic and able to socialize with ease with strangers, a typical TY type person also enjoys having the upper hand in relationships and tends to insist on having his own way. It is important to treat others with respect and to show kindliness and attentiveness. He is able to get through across to people, and while this skill of communication and penetration enables him to socialize easily with new people and mingle in with new acquaintances, he can also lack sufficient powers of discrimination and end up befriending people of treacherous, insidious nature. It would benefit him to heed carefully whom to put trust in and whom to socialize with.

Though clear-minded and creative, he tends to expect more than what the world is actually ready to offer him, and when he feels betrayed and disillusioned by the let-down or is faced with unanticipated setbacks, he can experience frustration and fury. Instead of getting down to solve the problem or dealing with the origin of the damage, he tends to phase into denial and resort to drinking, evading the real-life situations. The value of continued attentiveness and honest application should be understood.

The Soyang (SY) constitutional type persons usually have a strong sense of justice and are direct and straightforward. When they realize that they had been deceived and betrayed, they become depressed and dejected, which when prolonged can lead to lethargy and inertia. As a way of overcoming this, rearranging their home or making minor changes to the routine can allow them to start off again renewed and refreshed.

Though not shy to delve into new adventures and new projects, they often lack the tenacity to hold on at length and tend to give up in the middle. It is important to check before starting out whether they are capable of the task and whether they have the determination to finish the job.

Rather than seek real, substantial gain, they pursue glory and fame in the splendor of the world. They embellish and flaunt themselves, wanting to be held in high regard, perhaps more than they actually deserve. Developing one's assets and improving the self should take place before one rushes into action.

The typical SY type person can be a capable worker in the outside world, but back inside the house, he can be an unorganized and irresponsible caretaker for the family. Because the home and family together construct the basis for living, it would be wise to invest more energy into taking care of the household. His nimble, quick-witted quality allows him to excel at processing tasks, but his mercurial pursuit of splendor and attention to the outward appearances cause him to concentrate on adorning and embellishing himself, often leading to extravagance and arrogance. It is always wise to pursue only deserving appreciation and accept simplicity and temperance as a virtue.

The Taeeum (TE) constitutional type persons are known to lean toward inactivity, anticipating aid from the outside without making active efforts themselves. Their conservative nature resists changes, wanting to settle into the present state of things in the comforts of the familiar surroundings. It is important to expand oneself beyond the fences of the small world and experience the world, accumulate more knowledge, and broaden the scope of view. Personally exploring the world would be the most effective method, but if the chances are unavailable, second-hand experiences through reading, watching TV, watching movies, and so on can also serve as a gateway to the outside world.

Though they find venturing out on a new project and formulating new plans apprehensive and sometimes tiresome, having once taken on a task for themselves, being the strong, silent type with a patient nature, they are able to put continuous energy into it until the final completion. They are steadfast and reliable, generally taking good care of their home and family. However, because they can be less perceptive of the changes or new events in the outside world, they can be easily deceived or often find themselves placed in a difficult situation. It is advisable to always keep an eye open for what is really happening in the unfamiliar but nevertheless very real world. It is tempting to turn away from the hassle of interacting with strangers or learning of new things in life outside of the familiar and comfortable realm, but by giving in to the temptation, the TE-type person will eventually find himself caged inside a very small, narrow world. In this case, because he firmly believes that nothing exists outside the visible and tangible world, he also puts his value in the most material form of wealth and power in the present time, usually represented by money. Obsession with money can sometimes lead to acquisitive and possessive greed, and this should be overcome by experiencing the outside world and expanding one's knowledgeability.

The Soeum (SE) constitutional type persons are known for their genial, gentle, and tender personalities, with soft and warm heart, usually attentive and considerate of others, and these qualities attract a wide circle of friends. However, they secretly anticipate protection from the tight network of people, and such reliance on the system they have constructed or worked into should be discouraged, by always striving for self-sufficiency through actual, authentic efforts and actions.

Excessive diffidence and cautiousness are factors that urge the typical SE type person to opt for the safest choices in only winning situations. This need to have a sure footing can cause him to waste too much time planning and calculating and miss out on the crucial timing. He ought to be reminded that boldness can sometimes be the perfect solution. He often prefers to stay in the dark and strategize silently, but he needs to make sure that this is not based on self-serving calculations but rather for fair and honorable purposes. Because of his introverted and shy personality, he tends to associate with familiar people and flock together with friends, usually uncertain about making new acquaintances. However, socializing with new group of people can be beneficial and contribute to personal growth, and it is advisable to lose the apprehension and open up to new folks. He can also have small-hearted, jealous streaks, the grudge-bearing type who harbors age-old grievances, and because this can affect the body and cause illnesses, it should be overcome by learning to express the inner thoughts and emotions out into the open.

He has a soothing, placating effect on those around him, and this quality can attract and draw people. However, inside his heart resides an anticipation of being protected and taken care after by others, and he furtively yearns to infiltrate a secure, stable power system or gather sufficient clout. He may not be above obsessing over and abusing the power put into his hands, and vigilance is advised to remain alert and morally up-right.

The Doctrine of the Mean (Zhongyong 中庸), one of the four classical Confucian Canons (Sishu 四書 "Four Books"), mentions that "the unexpressed state of the emotions (joy, anger, sorrow, pleasure) is called Temperance (中), while the expressed but appropriate state of the emotions is called Harmony (和)." The ability to control the mind is not complete at the moment of birth, but is rather acquired by constant vigilance and retrospection of the joy, anger, sorrow, and pleasure in the mind. Disharmony of the body will rectify itself when the mind is successfully controlled.

3. Appropriate Exercises

The TE-type persons should select a high-intensity exercise. They need to consume and eliminate what they voraciously eat through dynamic activities. Because the TE-type persons tend to pay attention not only to their own personal matters but also to their physical bodies, they have excessive greed for food, which leads to the danger of becoming obese. Their obesity can be prevented through profuse sweating by doing sufficient exercises. It is a sign of health when the TE-type persons sweat profusely in daily life and it would be beneficial to their health if they could exercise regularly to sweat profusely.

It is recommended, therefore, to practice a heavy intensity exercise such as weight training or jogging for an extended time at a high speed to get a sufficient amount of exercise.

On the contrary, SE-type persons should be careful not to choose highly intense exercises. No matter what exercise is chosen, it will not improve their health if they do it to exhaustion. The people who stated that exercise is useless since exercising lowered their appetite and made them tired were most likely SE-type persons who exercised beyond their capabilities.

The SE-type persons are cautioned not to overwork themselves into exhaustion because they have constitutional weakness in their vital energy. Hence, it would be better to consider the state of their physical conditions and select exercises that do not require much energy. It is important for the SE-type persons to think of performing exercises that cover the entire body while maintaining a moderate amount of muscle tension, and developing their flexibility, rather than developing a steel-like body and big muscles through an exercise such as weight training. Exercises like calisthenics and jogging which do not overburden their bodies are recommended, as well as, quick and high intensity exercise such as tennis for a short time on regular basis. Even if it is not an exercise, the health cultivating activities that require much consumption of body energy, for example, a sauna, are likely to be only harmful for the SE-type persons.

The exercise intensity for both the TY and SY type lie in the middle range. That is, though they are not so weak in physical strength as the SE-type person, they need not sweat heavily every time like the TE-type persons.

Curriculum Vitae

Name: **Prof. Koh, Byung-Hee, M.D.(KM), Ph.D.**

Office Address: 1 Hoegi-dong, Dongdaemun-gu, Seoul, Korea
Dept. of Sasang Constitutional Medicine,
College of Korean Medicine, Kyung-Hee University,
Seoul, Korea
E-mail : kohbh@khu.ac.kr

Education

2005.8-2018.3	Chief Professor, Dept. of Sasang Constitutional Medicine, College of Korean Medicine, Kyung-Hee University
1998.9-2000.8	Visiting Professor, University of Bridgeport, CT. U.S.A.
1993.3-2005.8	Director of Dept. of Sasang Constitutional Medicine, Kyung-Hee University Medical Center
1982.3 –	Professor, Dept. of Constitutional Medicine, Kyung-Hee University Medical center
1983.9-1986.8	Kyung-Hee Graduate course of Oriental Medicine (Doctor)
1979.3-1981.2	Kyung-Hee Graduate course of Oriental Medicine (Master)
1973.3-1979.2	College of Oriental Medicine, Kyung-Hee University.

Academic Positions

2012.1 –	Convener, ISO TC249/WG5 (TCM Terminology & Informatics)
2012.8 –	Board Member, Society of Integrated Medicine
2012.8 –	Vice chairman, Society of Special Committee of Constitutional Medicine, WFCMS (World Federation of Chinese Medicine Societies)
2008.2-2018.3	Editor-in-chief, Journal of Sasang Constitutional Medicine.
2004.3-2009.3	Director, International Studies of Oriental Medicine, Kyunghee Univ.
2000.10-2003.10	President, Korea Institute of Oriental Medicine
1998.3-1998.8	Board Member, Society of Oriental Medicine
1996.4 –	Board Member, Society of Sasang Constitutional Medicine

1994.11-1997.2	Executive secretary, Institute of Oriental Med. Kyung-Hee Univ.
1994.4 –	Honorary President, Society of Information in Oriental Medicine
1994.4-1996.4	President, Society of Sasang Constitutional Medicine
1992.9-1994.4	President, Society of Information in Oriental Medicine
1991.8–	Honorary Board Member, Liaoning Society of Chinese Medicine
1991.9-1993.3	Inspector, Association of Oriental Medicine, Kyung-Hee Univ.
1990.3-1994.3	Executive Secretary, Society of Sasang Constitutional Medicine
1985.3-1990.3	Administrative manager, Society of Sasang Constitutional Medicine

- Koh Byung-Hee et el : Methodological Study for differentiating 5 Viceral Symptoms in Oriental Medicine, J. of East-West Medicine, 6:1, Jae-Han Institute of Oriental Medicine, 1981, pp.32-45.
- Koh Byung-Hee et el : Study of Heart Theory in Dr. Lee Jae-ma, J. of Association of Korean Oriental Medicine, 5:1, 1984, pp.39-44.
- Koh Byung-Hee et el: Bibliographical Study of five visceral deficiency Syndrome, J. of oriental pathology, 1, Society of Korean oriental pathology, 1984, pp.46-52.
- Koh Byung-Hee et el: Consideration for discerning Sa-sang Constitution, J. of AKOM, 6:1, 1985, pp.40-47.
- Koh Byung-Hee et el : An experimental study of Dear horn, Rehmania glutinosa, Panax Ginseng and Acanthopanax sessiliflorum on immune response and NK cell activity, J. of Kyung-Hee University, Vol. 9, 1986, pp.193-216.
- Song IB, Hong ND, Kim NJ, Koh BH et el: An experimental Study of Chung-hyul-ganggi-t'ang J. of Kyung-Hee University, 15, 1986, pp.163-172.
- Koh Byung-Hee et el: Immune Response and NK-cell activity of Antler, Rehmannia, Ginseng and Acanthopanax, J. of AKOM 7:2, AKOM 1986, pp.157-173.
- Koh Byung-Hee et el: The Oriental food therapy and Contraindication, Food and Nutrition, 7:4, The Bureau of Agricultural Development, 1986, pp.30-34.
- Koh Byung-Hee et el: An experimental Study of Sipimigwanjoongt'ang, J. of Oriental Med, 9, 1986, pp.437-450.
- Oh YS, Koh BH, Song IB et el : An experimental Study of 3 kinds of Ginseng in Immune response, J. of Kyung-Hee University Medical Center, 3:1, Kyung-Hee University Medical Center 1987, pp.82-90.
- Koh Byung-Hee et el: A methodology study of differential diagnosis of Sasang constitution, J of AKOM, 8:1, 1987, pp.139-145, pp.146-160.
- Hwang YM, Koh BH, Song IB et el: An experimental study of three

kinds of Rehmannia in Immune response, J. of Kyung-Hee University Medical Center, 3:3, 1987, pp.361-368.

- Koh Byung-Hee, Song I. B. : Characteristics of Sasang Constitutional Medicine, Abstract of International Symposium of East-West Medicine, Institute of Oriental Medicine, 1988, pp.187-192.
- Koh Byung-Hee et el: An experimental study of Kamigeopoongsan for Soeum Person, J. of Kyung-Hee University Medical Center, 4:1, 1988, pp.54-61.
- Koh Byung-Hee et el: An experimental study of Jeonhojihwangt'ang for Soyang Person, J. of Kyung-Hee University Medical Center, 4:4, 1988, pp.419-424.
- Cho HS, Koh BH, Song IB et el: An experimental study of Sunghyangjunggisan for Soeum Person, J. of Oriental Med of Kyung-Hee University, 11, 1988.
- Koh Byung-Hee et el: An experimental study of Hyungbangjihwangt'ang for Soyang Person, J. of Kyung-Hee University Medical Center, 5:2, 1989.
- Koh Byung-Hee, Kim Y. G, Song I. B : The psychosomatic aspect of D.M. in Sasang Constitutional Medicine, J. Constitutional Medicine, 1:1, society of Sasang Constitutional Medicine, 1989, pp.61-66.
- Koh Byung-Hee, Song I. B, Choi B. I : Application of acupuncture treatment in Sasang Constitutional Medicine , J. of Constitutional Medicine, 1:1, Society of Sasang Constitutional Medicine, 1989, pp.183-188.
- Koh Byung-Hee, Heo M. H., Song I. B. : The morphological study of Sasang Constitution, J. of Constitutional Medicine, 1:1, 1989, pp.29-40.
- Kim SB, Koh BH, Song IB : Study for establishing the database in classification of Sasang constitution, J. of Oriental Med of Kyung-Hee University, 12, 1989.
- Koh Byung-Hee, Jang H. J, Song I. B. : Consideration about Soeum Person's symptom, J of AKOM, 11:1, 1990.

- Koh Byung-Hee, Han. J. S, Song I. B. : An experimental study of Galgeunhaekit'ang for Taeum Person in immune response and NK cell Activity, J. of AKOM, 11:2, 1990.
- Koh Byung-Hee, Song I. B, Choi B. I. : The Basic theory and background of Dr. Lee Jaema, J. of Constitutional Medicine, 2:1, 1990, pp.23-46.
- Koh Byung-Hee, Kim D. R., Song I. B. : Study for academic resources and the developing period of Dr. Lee Jaema's theory, J. of Constitutional Medicine, 2:1, 1990, pp. 1-22.
- Koh Byung-Hee. Song J. M., Song I. B. : Study of four cosmology in Sung-Myung chapter, J. of Constitutional Medicine, 2:1, 1990, pp.47-56
- Koh Byung-Hee, Heo M. H., Song I. B. : Study for understanding Hwak-Choong Chapter, J. of Constitutional Medicine, 2:1, 1990, pp.57-70.
- Koh Byung-Hee, Kim J. W., Song I. B., : Consideration of visceral theory in Sasang Constitutional Medicine, J. of Constitutional Medicine, 2:1, 1990, pp.87-102.
- Koh Byung-Hee, Kim S. B., Song I. B., : Bibliographical study on mechanism and treatment of Dam-Eum(Sputum or expectoration) in Sasang Constitutional Medicine, J. of Constitutional Medicine, 1990, pp.103-114.
- Koh Byung-Hee, Song I. B., : An experimental study of four kinds of antler in Immune response, J. of Kyung-Hee University, 9, 1990.
- Koh Byung-Hee, Kim J. H., Song I. B., : Consideration of Nature and Emotion in the cosmology of Dr. Lee Jaema, J. of Oriental Med of Kyung-Hee University, 13, 1990.
- Koh Byung-Hee, Kim, Jang H. J., Song I. B., : Study of personal deed and understanding of human being, J. of Constitutional Medicine, 3:1, 1991, pp.23-34.
- Koh Byung-Hee, Cho H. S., Song I. B., : Study of Yuryak Chapter in Kyukchigo, J. of Constitutional Medicine, 3:1, 1991, pp.35-66.

- Koh Byung-Hee, Kim J. W., Analysis of 53 admitted patients through QSCC, J. of Constitutional Medicine, 3:1, 1991, pp.89-104.
- Koh Byung-Hee, Han J. S., Song I. B., Theory of longevity in Dongeuisoosebowon and Jaejoongsinp'yun, J. of Constitutional Medicine, 3:1, 1991, pp.141-150.
- Koh Byung-Hee, Basic theory of Sasang Constitutional Medicine, J. of practical Internal Medicine in Chinese Medicine, 6:1, Institute of Liaoning Chinese Medicine, 1992, pp.1-4./J. of Constitutional Medicine, 4:1, 1992, p.77.
- Koh Byung-Hee, Cho B. G., Masao S, Skin conductance level in four constitution, ,J. Medical Engineering, 30, Japanese society of Medical Engineering, 1992, pp.619./ J. of Constitutional Medicine, 4:1, 1992, p.187.
- Koh Byung-Hee, Moon S. H., Song I. B., : An experimental study of Jaejo in thrombosis, J. of Kyung-Hee University Medical Center, 8:2, 1992, pp.177.
- Koh Byung-Hee, Jo H. S., Song I. B., : Study on Yuryak Chapter in Kyukchigo, J. of Constitutional Medicine, 4:1, 1992, pp.31.
- Koh Byung-Hee, Cheun E. Y., Kim G. B., : Study on healthy condition about stress recognition according to constitution in Korean, J. of Constitutional Medicine, 4:1, 1992, pp.81.
- Koh Byung-Hee, Heo M. H., Song J. M., Kim D. R., : A Morphological Study on Sasang Constitution, Heo M. H., J. of Constitutional Medicine, 4:1, 1992, pp.107.
- Koh Byung-Hee, Lee J. C., Song I. B., : Comparative study on Validity between QSCC And 6-PF Payroll nature factor test, 7nd ICOM Seminar, International association of Oriental Medicine in Taiwan, 1992.
- Koh Byung-Hee, Kim S. H., Song I. B., : Validation Study on QSCC, 2nd International Seminar of Oriental Medicine, 2, International association of Oriental Medicine in Taiwan, 1992, pp. 182.
- Koh Byung-Hee et el : Variation of Heart Rate and the Densities of

Sodium and Potassium in Serum According to the Physical Constitution, 7th, International Congress on Biomedical Engineering, International Society of Bio-engineering, Singapore, 1992, pp.570.

- Byung ill Choi, Byung hee Koh and Il Byuung Song : Effects of Soyangin-yanggueksanwhatang, indongdeungjigolpitang and sook-jiwhanggosamtang on the Alloxan-Induced diabetic Rats, J. Kyunghee Ori. Med. Vol. 15, pp.113~133, 1992.
- Koh Byung-Hee : Modern Application of Traditioal Medicine, Searching Our Culture, Central Education Institute of National Government, 1993, pp.3-41.
- Koh Byung-Hee : Study on Personality Analysis with 16 Personality Factor in Sasang Constitution, J of AKOM, 14:2, 1993, pp.64 76.
- Koh Byung-Hee, Jo B. K., Bae Jong I. L., Masao S,: Study of Acid-Base balance and difference in pulse rate and electrorites level according to Constitution, J of AKOM, 14:2, 1993, pp.320-326.
- Koh Byung-Hee, Park B. K., Song J. Y., Lee J. H., Jang H. I., Jeon S. I., : A Study on the application of the Constitutional Model Originated by Je-Ma Lee to the Somatic Symptoms of the Patients with Somatoform Disorders, J. of the Korean Neuropsychiatric Association, 32:6, Korean Neuropsychiatric Association, 1993, pp.863-885.
- Koh Byung-Hee, Hong J. H., : A Study of Taehak and Joongyong in Kyukchigo, J. of Constitutional Medicine, 5:1, 1993, pp.41-54.
- Kim Sun-ho, Koh Byung-Hee, Song I. B., : Validative Studies of Sasang Constitution Classification Questionnaire, J. of Constitutional Medicine, 5:1, 1993, p.61.
- Koh Byung-Hee, Lee J. C., Song I. B., : Validative Studies of Sasang Constitution Classification, J. of Constitutional Medicine, 5:1, 1993, pp.87-104.
- Koh Byung-Hee, Song I. B., Kim J. W., Kim J. W., : Comparative study on constitutional diagnosis and personal characteristics analysing QSCC and MMPI, J. of AKOM, 15:1 1994. pp.66-74.

- Koh Byung-Hee : Sasang Constitution and General Management of Life, The 1st International conference on Health Care, 1994. pp.25-33 Muju Resort curing lab.
- Koh Byung-Hee; Present Condition of Sasang Constitution in Korea, Journal of the first Sasang Medicine international conference, 1994.8.5. pp.1-9.
- Jo YT, Koh BH, Song I. B ; A Study on Norm Validation in the Questionnaire for the Sasang Constitution Classification, Journal of the first Sasang Medicine international conference 1994.8.5. pp.65-91.
- Koh BH, Kwon YJ; The role of Oriental Medicine in School, 1994 Textbook of Nursing Teacher Education, Seoul Office of School Health Management, 1994.10.18. pp.27-117.
- Koh BH, Cho YT, Song IB; Validation Study of the QSCC (comparative Study with 16PF and MBTI); International Symposium on East-West Medicine 1994.10.20 pp.56-57. Sheraton Walker Hill Hotel, Seoul, Korea/J. of Constitutional Medicine, 6:1, p.21, 1994.
- Koh BH; Objective approach for Sasang Constitution Classification ; 17th National Seminar of Oriental Medicine paper abstracts, pp.10-21, 1994.10.23. Lotte Hotel.
- Cho HS, Koh BH, Song IB ; An experimental Study of several medicinal formulas for Soeum and Soyang Person on Hyperthyroidism ; 17th J. of Oriental Med. of Kyung-Hee University, 1994.8.15. pp.201-223.
- Kim JW, Koh BH, Song IB: 「A Study of Chapter Dokhang(Personal Deed)」, J Sasang Constitute Med. 4:1, 1994, pp 95-116.
- Kim JY, Koh BH, Song IB, : 「A Study of Knowledge and Deed in Sasang Constitutional Medicine(Dockhaengphyeon, Seongmyeongron, Sadanron)」, J Sasang Constitute Med.7:1, 1995, pp1-6.
- Kim JW, Koh BH, Song IB; 「A Study of The Correlativity in EAV(Electroacupuncture According to Voll) measurement values, Sasang Constitution Classification and CVA(Cerebrovascular acci-

dent)」, 8th Journal of ICOM, 1995, pp89-91,248-249. ,/ J Sasang Constitute Med. 7:2, 1995, p.59.

- Lee EJ, Koh BH, Song IB: The Study on The Validity of "Questionnaire of Sasang Constitution Classification(I), 8th Journal of ICOM, 1995, pp286,202., J Sasang Constitute Med. 7:2, 1995, p.89.
- Jung BY, Koh BH, Song IB: Bibliographical Study of Medicinal Herbs in Constitutional Medicine, J Sasang Constitute Med. 7:1, 1995, pp135-180.
- Song JM, Song IB, Koh BH: An experimental Study of several Herb Formula for Taeum and Soeum Person on the effect of Autonomic Nerve system, J Sasang Constitute Med. 7:1, 1995, pp183-213.
- An KM, Song IB, Koh BH: An experimental Study of Bojoongikgit'ang on the Effect of Yang Deficiency Syndrome, 8th Journal of ICOM, 1995, pp283-284,198-199.
- Hong SC, Koh BH, Song IB: An experimental Study of Chungsimyonjat'ang for Taeum Person, 8th Journal of ICOM, 1995, pp282,196-197. /J. Sasang Constitute Med. 7:2, 1995, p.227.
- Lee SK, Koh BH, Song IB: Bibliographical Study of Various Syndrome in Taeum Person, J Sasang Constitute Med. 7:2, 1995, pp103-116.
- Lee EJ, Koh BH, Song IB : Consideration of Constitutional Food, J Sasang Constitute Med. 7:2, 1995, pp143-168.
- Jung BY, Koh BH, Song IB: Bibliographical Study of Medicinal Herbs in Constitutional Medicine, J Sasang Constitute Med. 7:2, 1995, pp135.
- Kim JY, Koh BH, Song IB, Kim JW: Classification and Application of Constitutional Food, J Sasang Constitute Med. 7:2, 1995, pp263-280.
- Jang YK, Koh BH, Song IB: An experimental Study of Sibjundaebot'ang for Soeum Person on the effect of Yang Deficiency Syndrome, 8th Journal of ICOM, 1995, pp285,200-201./ J Sasang Constitute Med.

7:1, 1995, p.281.

- Koh BH: Application of Acupuncture in Constitutional Medicine WFAS' 95 Symposium on Acupuncture & QI, 1995, Istanbul-Turkey, 1995, p 40.
- Koh BH et al; Morphological study for objectification of Sasang constitutional diagnosis, Art Anatomical Institute, 1996.
- Koh Byung-Hee et al : A Morphological Study on Head and Face according to the Sa-Sang Constitution, J. of Oriental Medicine, Institute of Oriental Medicine, 1:.1 1996. 12. 20.
- Koh BH, Cho YJ, Choi CS, Kim JW, Hong SC, Song IB: A Morphological Study on Head and Face according to the Sa-Sang Constitution, 2nd Journal of Sasang medicine international conference,pp.27-34,1996.8.7.America LA Harvard Grand Hotel.
- Koh BH: An Introduction of Sasang Constitutional Medicine, The 6th International Conference of Oriental Medicine, pp.1-16. 1996. 8. 9. America Las Vegas Hacienda Hotel.
- Koh BH, Yoon DY: Consideration of 4 wicked-minded person in Chapter Dokhang in Kyukchigo, J Sasang Constitute Med,8:1, 1996.8. pp.57-74.
- Koh BH, Song IB, Cho YJ, Choi CS, Hong SC, Lee EJ, Lee SR, Seo JS: A Morphological Study on Head and Face according to the Sa-Sang Constitution, J Sasang Constitute Med.8:1, 1996.8, pp.101-186.
- Koh BH, Kim SH, Song IB: A Study for Standardization of QSCC(II), J Sasang Constitute Med. 7:1, 1995 p.187 / 8:1, 1996. pp.187-246.
- Koh BH, Lee JC, Song IB: Validative Study of QSCC(II), J Sasang Constitute Med. 8:1, 1996. 8. pp.247-294.
- Koh BH, Lee SK, Lee EJ, Hong SC: An Analysis on the Characteristics of Sa-Sang Constitution, J Sasang Constitute Med. 8:1, 1996. 8. pp.349-376.
- Koh BH, Kim JY: Rudimentary Presentation on Menu for Diabetes

(1800kcal) in Taeumin, Soumin, and Soyangin based on Food Lists by Constitution, J Sasang Constitute Med. 8:1 1996. 8. pp.395-412.

- Koh BH, Kim SH, Song IB: A Study for Standardization of QSCC(II), 18th Journal of National Korean medicine conference, 1996.11.9.pp.268-331/ /J Sasang Constitute Med. 7:1 1995. p.187.
- Koh BH, Lee EJ, Song IB: An analysis on the characteristic of phisical examination, Journal of Korean Medicine in Geriatric diseases 2:1 1996. 11. pp.48-62.
- Kim IT, Koh BH, Song IB: The comparison study of the structure of mind and psychological type of C.G Jung to Ji-In-Lon and Sa-Sang constitution of Lee Je Ma, J Sasang Constitute Med. 8:2, 1996.
- Cha CJ, Lee SR, Lee EJ, Hong SC, Kim JW, Koh BH, Song IB: A Study on the standardization of EAV(Electroacupuncture acc. Voll)'s measurement values, J Sasang Constitute Med. 8:2 1996.
- Cho DW, Lee CS, Koh BH, Cho HS; Genetic Analysis Study of Sasang Constitution Classification by DNA-fingerprinting methods, J Sasang Constitute Med. 8:2 1996.
- Cho MS, Koh BH; Review of menopause in Sasang constitutional medicine, J Sasang Constitute Med. 8:2 1996.
- Noh SH, Lee EJ, Hong SC, Koh BH, Song IB: The Study on the Validity of "Questionnaire of Sasang Constitution Classification", J Sasang Constitute Med. 8:2 1996.
- Hong SC, Koh BH, Song IB; A study on The manuscripts left by Dong-Mu for the chronological table of Lee Jae-Ma, Korean Journal of Oriental Medicine Vol.2.1996.
- Cho HS, Koh BH, Lee CS, Hong SC, Lee EJ, Kwon GH, Cho DW; Genetic analysis study of Sasang Constitution classification, Korean Journal of Oriental Medicine Vol.2.1996.
- Koh BH, Cho YJ, Choi CS, Hong SC, Kim JW, Lee EJ, Lee SY, Seo JS, Song IB ; A Morphological Study on Head and Face according to the Sa-Sang Constitution, Journal of Oriental Medicine, Institute of Oriental Medicine, 1:1 1996. 12. 20.

- Eui-Ju Lee, Byunghee Koh, Il Byung Song, ; An Analysis on the characteristics of physical examination – centering on the groups dividen by obesity score, J. of Oriental chr. dis. 2:1, 1996.
- Koh BH; TaeGuk Acupuncture, Journal of the 2nd European Acupuncture Conference,1997.05.28.
- Koh BH; Standardization of EAV measurement Value, Journal of the 2nd European Acupuncture Conference,1997.05.28.
- Sung SJ, Song IB, Koh BH et al; According to Sa-Sang constitution, the investigation of numerical value of measurement about Yang-do-rack diagnosis, J. of Oriental Med of Kyung-Hee University, 1997. 07.15.
- Koh BH et al; The effects of Galgunhaegit`ang and Won`s-Galgunhaegit`ang for Taeumin on the immune response, J Sasang Constitute Med. 9:1, 1997. 08.30.
- Koh BH; The Eumyang Standpoint in Physiological and Pathological Phenomena in Sasang Constitutional Medicine, J Sasang Constitute Med. 9:1, 1997. 08.30.
- Koh BH; A Morphologic Study of head and face for Sasang Constitution, J Sasang Constitute Med., 9:2 1997.10.07.
- Koh BH; Objectification research of Sasang constitutional diagnosis by genetic analysis, Korea Institute of Oriental Medicine, 3rd Journal of Korea Institute of Oriental Medicine conference, 1997.11.22. J Sasang Constitute Med. 9:2 1997, p.147.
- Koh BH; Translation of Dongmuyugo, Journal of 1st International Korean medicine conference, Institute of Oriental Medicine, KyungHee University, 1997.11.26.
- Koh BH et al; Clinical study on the effect of Ginseng on the healthy person's constitution, Research Service Report, Kyung Hee University, Korea Ginseng and Tobacco Research Institute, 1997.12.31.
- Koh BH et al; Genetic Analysis of Sasang Constitution by Amp-FLP Method, J Sasang Constitute Med. 9:2 1997, p.163.
- Koh BH et al; The Bibliographical Investigation of the Apple and

Neung-keum, Journal of Korean Oriental Medicine, 1998. 04.01.

- Koh BH et al; A Study on the Appropriate Herbal Medicine According to Sasang Constitution Using EAV, The 9th ICOM Abstract, 1998. 07. 24.
- Koh BH et al; Morphological study for objectification of Sasang constitutional diagnosis, J Sasang Constitute Med. 10:1, 1998. 08.31, p.171.
- Koh BH et al; A Study on the morphologic characteristics of each Constitution`s trunk, J Sasang Constitute Med. 10:1, 1998. 08.31, p.101.
- Koh BH et al; Philological study on Sasang constitutional medicine's formation process, J Sasang Constitute Med. 10:1, 1998. 08.31, p.41.
- Koh BH et al; Sasang Constitutional Medicine and Health Management, Association of Korean Medicine International Medical Corps, 1998.08.31.
- Koh BH et al; Clinical study on the effect of Ginseng on the healthy person's constitution, Journal of the 2nd Korean medical center conference.1998.09.12.
- Koh BH et al; The effects of proliferation and differentiation on adipocyte 3T3-L1 by herbs and herbal prescriptions of Soeumin and Soyangin, Institute of Korean Medicine in Kyung Hee University Korean medicine, 1998. 11. 27.
- Koh BH et al; The Characteristics of the Viscera and Bowels of Sasang Constitutional Medicine, Journal of Oriental medicine, 1998. 12.31.
- Hong SC, Koh BH, Song IB et al; A Morphologic Study of Ear, Eye, Nose and Mouth according to the Sasang Constitution, J Sasang Constitute Med.1998. 12. 31.
- Koh BH et al; A Morphologic Study On The Upper Face of Moiré According to the Sasang Constitution, J Sasang Constitute Med. 1998. 12.31.

- Koh BH et al; A clinical study on the constitutional characteristics of diabetes mellitus patients, J. of Oriental Chronic Disease, 1998. 12.31.
- Koh BH et al; The Clinical Study of the Constitutional Characteristics of the Fatty Liver Patients, Kyung hee medicine. 1998. 12.31.
- Koh BH et al; The Bibliographical Investigation of effect of Clematis mandshurica Maxim, J Sasang Constitute Med. 1998. 12.31.
- Koh BH et al; A Morphologic Study of Sasang Constitution, J Sasang Constitute Med, 1998. 12.31.
- Koh BH et al; Reference Consideration for corn, J Sasang Constitute Med, 1998. 12.31.
- Koh BH et al; Treatment case on carbuncle and cellulitis of Soyangin, J Sasang Constitute Med, 1998. 12.31.
- Kim SB, Koh BH, Song IB et al; The effects of proliferation and differentiation on adipocyte 3T3-L1 by prescriptions and Taeyang-In and Taeum-In, J Sasang Constitute Med, 1998. 12.31.
- Cho MS, Koh BH, Song IB et al; A Clinical Study of the Obesity Patients according to Sasang Constitution, J Sasang Constitute Med, 10:2, 1998.
- Koh BH et al; The Study of Constitutional Dietary Therapy, J Sasang Constitute Med, 10:2, 1998, p.305.
- Koh BH et al; The Bibliographical investigation of effect of Acorus gramineus Soland, J Sasang Constitute Med, 1999.
- Koh BH et al; The Bibliographical investigation of the mallow, hollyhock, darkpull, sunflower, J Sasang Constitute Med, 1999.
- Koh BH et al; The study on the structure of the Lee Je-ma`s viewpoint of Morpho-Image, J Sasang Constitute Med,1999.
- Koh BH et al; A Clinical Study of the Constitutional Therapeutic Diet Plan, Kyung Hee Medicine, 2000.
- Koh BH et al; The Bibliographical investigation of effect of GYPSUM FIBROSUM in Dongyi Soose Bowon, J Sasang Constitute Med, 2000.

- Lee JH, Koh BH, Song IB et al; The Clinical Study on the Constitutional symptomatic pattern of Soyangin and Taeumin in-patients in stroke, J Sasang Constitute Med, 2000.
- Koh BH et al; The Combination of the Traditional and the Modern Medicine in Korea: Trends and Perspectives, Journal of International conference in Kyung Hee medical center Opening of the 30th anni versary, 2001.
- Lee SK, Lee EJ, Kim SB, Koh BH, Song IB et al; A study on the validity to make a diagnosis of Soeumin by QSCC Ⅱ(Questionnaire for Sasang Constitution Classification Ⅱ), J Sasang Constitute Med, 2000.
- Lee SK, Lee EJ, Yoon JH, Song IB, Koh BH et al; Morphological standardization research of head and face on the 50's and 60's in Korean according to Sasang Constitution, J Sasang Constitute Med, 2000.
- Lim KS, Kim SB, Lee JH, Park GS, Lee SK, Lee EJ, Yoon JH, Koh BH, Song IB et al; The Comparison Research of the Head and Face on the 30's, 40's, and the 50's, 60's in Korean Men according to Sasang Constitution, J Sasang Constitute Med, 2000.
- Koh BH et al; A Study on the validity to make a diagnosis of Taeumin by QSCCII(Questionnaire for the Sasang Constitution Classification), J Sasang Constitute Med, 2001.
- Koh BH et al; The Clinical Study on the Body Weight Loss of Taeumin Inpatients on Stroke by Sasang Constitutional Medicinal Treatment, J Sasang Constitute Med, 2001.
- Lee EJ, Lim JH, Koh BH, Song IB et al; Comparison With `Gu-Bon` and 'in-Bon' on Symptom of Soemin`s Disease and Soyangin`s Disease, J Sasang Constitute Med, 2001.
- Koh BH et al; A study on `the Discourse on the Constitutional Symptoms and Disease` of 『Dongyi Soose Bowon』 written in 1894, J Sasang Constitute Med, 2001.
- Koh BH et al; The 21st Century Medical Revolution and Oriental

Medicine, The 21st Century Medical Revolution and Oriental Medicine, 2001.

- Koh BH et al; Oriental medical strategies according to China's WTO accession, Healthcare International Cooperation Strategy Development Seminar, Department of Health and Human Services, 2001.
- Koh BH et al; A Case of Treatment of a Taeumin patient with Sweaty Scrotum and Dysuria, J Sasang Constitute Med, 2001.
- Koh BH et al; The Clinical Study on the Effect of Sasang Constitutional Medical Therapy for Taeumin Patients in acute stroke. -, J Sasang Constitute Med, 2001.
- Koh BH et al; Soyangin mangeum-disease case study, J Sasang Constitute Med, 2001.
- Lee JH, Park KS, Koh BH et al; A Case Report on 'fever of unknown origin, abdominal distension and diarrhea' of Taeumin, J Sasang Constitute Med, 2001.
- Koh BH et al; A study on the correlation between Sasang Constitution and HLA type, J Sasang Constitute Med, 2002.
- Huh MH, Koh BH, Song IB et al; The Body Measuring Method to Classify to Sasang Constitutions, J Sasang Constitute Med, 2002.
- Lee EJ, Koh BH, Lim JH, Song IB et al; A study on the formative process of Taeumin prescription, J Sasang Constitute Med, 2002.
- Lee EJ, Koh BH, Lim JH, Song IB et al; A Study on Dong-mu's `Knowing and Acting`, J Sasang Constitute Med, 2002.
- Lee SK, Lee EJ, Jung YJ, Koh BH, Song IB et al; A study of preservation of health in the 「Dongyi Bogam」 and 「Dongyi Soose Bowon Sasang Chobongwon」, J Sasang Constitute Med, 2002.
- Kim SH, Kim HJ, Hong JM, Yoon YS, Koh BH, Choi SM et al; A study on the correlation between Sasang constitution and IL-4 polymorphism, J Sasang Constitute Med, 2002
- Koh BH et al; Direction and conditions of the globalization of Oriental Medicine, Proceedings of the International Symposium on Oriental Medicine modernization and globalization, Gyeongsan

University, 2002.
- Yu JH, Lee EJ, Koh BH, Song IB et al; The Study on the Upgrade of QSCC II (I) - A Study on Comparison of responses to the questionnaire based on Sasang constitution's differences-Questionnaire of Sasang Constitution Classification II (QSCCII), J Sasang Constitute Med, 2003.
- Kwak CG, Lee SK, Lee EJ, Koh BH, Song IB et al; The Study on the Upgrade of QSCC II (II) - The study on the re-validity of QSCC II, J Sasang Constitute Med, 2003.
- Koh BH et al; The bibliographical Investigation of songback(松栢), J Sasang Constitute Med, 2003.
- Koh BH et al; A case of Drug Eruptions of Soyangin patient mistreated with Taeumin, J Sasang Constitute Med, 2003.
- Lee EJ, Lim JH, Koh BH, Song IB et al; The Study about Dong-mu's Thought on Human in 『Dongyi Suse Bowon Sasang Choboguon』, J Sasang Constitute Med, 2003.
- Lee JG, Lim JH, Koh BH, Song IB et al; A Study on `Health` concept of Sasang Constitutional Medicine, J Sasang Constitute Med, 2003.
- Noh SH, Lee SK, Lee EJ, Koh BH, Song IB et al; A clinical study of Rheumatoid Arthritis prescribed Taeeumin Jowiseungchungtang, J Sasang Constitute Med, 2003.
- Kim IJ, Lee SK, Lee EJ, Koh BH, Song IB et al; The Sasang Constitutional Thought of Pulse Diagnosis, J Sasang Constitute Med, 2003.
- Kim SB, Lee SK, Lee EJ, Choi SM, Koh BH, Song IB, Jung YJ et al; Revision of the Questionnaire for the Sasang Constitution Classification, J Sasang Constitute Med, 2003.
- Koh BH et al; The Study on the Upgrade of QSCC II - The study on the re-validity of QSCCII-, 5th Sasang medicine International conference,2003.
- Ha MS, Koh BH, Song IB et al; A study on the correlation between Sasang Constitution and HLA type, 5th Sasang medicine International

conference,20030721.

- Koh BH et al; Perception and ways of coping with stress of Sasangin, 5th Sasang medicine International conference, 2003.
- Koh BH; Present and future of Ethnic Medicine, 2003 Ethnic Medicine conference South Korean Journal published, 2003.
- Koh BH et al; Sasang medicine challenges and prospects, 2nd Bukyoung University herbal medicine improvement Institute Symposium, 2004.
- Koh BH et al; A Case of Treatment of a Taeumin Patient diagnosed to Adrenoleukodystrophy, J Sasang Constitute Med, 2004.
- Koh BH et al; A Study on the Pharmacology of Sasang Constitutional Medicine, J Sasang Constitute Med, 2004.
- Koh BH et al; A Case of Taeumin diagnosed to Pleural effusion, J Sasang Constitute Med, 2004.
- Koh BH et al; Introduction of Constitutional medicine and management, Oriental Music Therapy Forum, Kunsan National University of Arts, 2004.
- Koh BH et al; A Study on Inclination of Mind and Nature & Emotion of Sasang Constitutional Medicine, J Sasang Constitute Med, 2004.
- Koh BH et al; A Study for Sasang Structure about 『Dongyi Suse Bowon』 and 『Gyukchigo』, J Sasang Constitute Med, 2004.
- Koh BH et al; A Study on the degree and Types of Gastritis and Gastrointestinal Symptoms according to Sasang Constitution and Gender Difference, J Sasang Constitute Med, 2004.
- Koh BH et al; Study for the mechanism of exterior, interior disease by the nature and emotion, J Sasang Constitute Med, 2004.
- Koh BH et al; A case of Moxibustion at Kil for a Soyangin patient with Insomnia, J Sasang Constitute Med, 2004.
- Koh BH et al; A Study about Construction of Sasang Constitutional Nursing Theory: On the focus 『Dongyi Soose Bowon Sasang Chobongwon』, J Sasang Constitute Med, 2004.

- Koh BH et al; What is alternative medicine, Korean medicine association the 7thPlannedSeminar, 2004.
- Koh BH; The Role of Oriental Medicine in the 21st Century, 4thTWGHs-CUHK Eddie Wang Symposium on Complementary Chinese and Western Medicine-, Hong Kong Baptist University, 20040227.
- Koh BH; Guidelines of the Medical Record, WHO Traditional medicine Standard treatment Guidelines Setting Expert conference, Seoul National University Natural Products Research Institute W.H.O. Traditional Oriental drugs Research Center, 2004.
- Koh BH et al; Sasang Constitutional Medicine in Korea, 20041130.
- Koh BH et al; Education in Oriental Medicine in KyungHee University, Evidence-based Complementary and Alternative Medicine, Oxford University Press, 2004.
- Kwak CG, Son EH, Yu JH, Koh BH, Song IB, Lee EJ et al; Research and Development of Herbal Medicine (Taeumbiman-tang) on Obesity, Korean Journal of Oriental Physiology and Pathology, 2005.
- Hwang MW, Lee SK, Choi BG, Song IB, Koh BH et al; The Research on the Sasang Constitutional Characteristics of Stroke Inpatients, J Sasang Constitute Med, 2005.
- Koh BH et al; Multicenter Cohort Collaboration for the Korean genome epidemiology, Services research and development project report, 2005.
- Lee JH, Lee SK, Lee EJ, Koh BH, Song IB et al; A Study on 「Gyukchigo. Yuryak」, J Sasang Constitute Med, 2005.
- Koh BH et al; A study on the Change of Conception about Soeumin Hwangdal(jaundice) between 「Dongyi Soose Bowon」 'GaboBon' and 'SinchukBon', J Sasang Constitute Med, 2005.
- Koh BH et al; A study on 'The Discourse on the Soeumin Gwakran Disease' of Dongmu Lee Je-Ma, J Sasang Constitute Med, 2005.
- Koh BH et al; A Case Study of Soeumin Jaundice Patient Diagnosed as Drug-Induced Hepatitis, J Sasang Constitute Med, 2005.

- Koh BH et al; A Case Study about Soyangin Patient suffering from Nausea and Vomiting, treated with Soyangin Superficial Disease, J Sasang Constitute Med, 2005.
- Son EH, Yu JH, Kim JW, Kim GG, Koh BH, Lee EJ, Song IB et al; The Study of Sasangin's Face, J Sasang Constitute Med, 2005.
- Koh BH et al; A Study on the Distributional Rate of Sasangin in Korea, J Sasang Constitute Med, 2005.
- Koh BH; The Roles of Sasang Constitutional Medicine in 21st Century, 6th Sasang constitutional medicine article abstracts, Sasang constitutional medicine, Korean Oriental Medical Society, 2005.
- Yu JH, Song IB, Baik SY, Koh BH, Lee EJ et al; Clinical Trial of Herbal Formula on weight Loss in Obese Korean Children, The American Journal of Chinese Medicine, World Scientific Publishing Company, 2005.
- Lee TG, Hwang MW, Ham TI, Lee SK, Choi BG, Koh BH, Song IB et al; A study on the Distributional Rate of Sasangin in Korea, The 13th International Congress of Oriental Medicine, The international Society of Oriental Medicine, The Association of Korean Oriental Medicine, 2005.
- Koh BH et al; The Case-control Study of ischemic Stroke According to Sasang Constitution, The 13th International Congress of Oriental Medicine, The International Society of Oriental Medicine, The Association of Korean Oriental Medicine, 2005.
- Koh BH et al; ,The Study on the effect of Oriental Music Therapy in ischemic stroke patients Classified by Sasang Constitutional Medicine, The 13th International Congress of Oriental Medicine, The International Society of Oriental Medicine, The Association of Korean Oriental Medicine, 20051022.
- Koh BH et al; Building DB for three-dimensional constitution diagnostic development, Health care technology promotion projects Annual/Stage performance. Plan, 2006.

- Choi KJ, Choi YS, Cha JH, Hwang MW, Lee Sk, Koh BH, Song IB et al; A study on the Reliability and Validity test of the QSCC2 (Revised Questionnaire for the Sasang Constitution Classification), J Sasang Constitute Med, 2006.
- Yu JH, Ahn SW, Lee EJ, Song IB, Koh BH et al; A Study about Construction of Sasang Constitutional Nursing Theory II – On the Focus of 『Dongyi Suse Bowon』 written in 1894 (Old Edition), J Sasang Constitute Med, 2006.
- Ko WS, Kim KS, Koh BH, Lee EJ et al; The Study on Sasangin's Characteristics of Elementary School Students, J Sasang Constitute Med, 2006.
- Hwang YM, Yu YB, Kim JY, Koh BH, Lee EJ et al; HPLC Analysis of Marker Substances in Taeumin Gamijowi-tang, J Sasang Constitute Med, 2006.
- Lee SK, Song IB, Koh BH, Kim HG et al; A Clinical Study on Sasang Constitutional Medical Treatment Effectiveness of Allergic Rhinitis Patients in Taeumin, J Sasang Constitute Med, 2006.
- Koh BH et al; An Positioning Error Analysis of 3D Face Recognition Apparatus, J Sasang Constitute Med, 2006.
- Koh BH et al; An Error Examination of 3D Face Automatic Recognition, J Sasang Constitute Med, 2006.
- Koh BH et al; A Study on the Reliability of the Questionnaire about Sasang Constitution Classification for Mongolians, J Sasang Constitute Med, 2006.
- Koh BH et al; The Study of Face Model and Face Type, J Sasang Constitute Med, 2006.
- Koh BH et al; A Case Study about Taeumin Patient Suffering from Nausea and Vomiting, Treated with Taeumin 'Interior-hot Disease', J Sasang Constitute Med, 2006.
- Koh BH et al; The Study on the Effect of Oriental Music Therapy in Ischemic Stroke Patients Classified by Sasang Constitutional Medicine, J Sasang Constitute Med, 2006.

- Koh BH et al; Research Report on Health Promotion for traditional medicine in Mongolia and South Korea diagnostic technology exchange and building, health promotion for traditional medicine in Mongolia and South Korea diagnostic technology exchange and build, KIOM ,2006.
- Koh BH et al; A Cohort Study of Sasang Constitutional Medicine, Academic services business report, Centers for Disease Control and Prevention, 2006.
- Koh BH et al; Precision Test of 3D Face Automatic Recognition Apparatus (3D-FARA) by Rotation, J Sasang Constitute Med, 2006.
- Koh BH et al; A Hardware Error Analysis of 3D Face Automatic Recognition Apparatus(3D-FARA), J Sasang Constitute Med, 2006.
- Koh BH et al; Methods of developing the Sasang constitutional discriminant function when the sample sizes vary greatly between the constitutional types, 18th annual AAMA symposium and the ICMART XII medical acupuncture congress, The American Academy of Medical Acupuncture, 20060408.
- Koh BH et al; An error analysis of 3D Face Recognition, journal of Japanese academy of facial studies, 20060930.
- Koh BH et al; A clinical study on SCM treatment effectiveness for allergic rhinitis patients, 15th congress of the European academy of dermatology and venereology, the European academy of dermatology and venereology, 20061006.
- Koh BH et al; A Study on the Concordance Rate of the Diagnostic Results Among Sasang Constitutional Medicine(SCM) Specialists, J Sasang Constitute Med, 2006.
- Koh BH et al; Point Recognition Precision Test of 3D Automatic Face Recognition Apparatus(3D-AFRA), J Sasang Constitute Med, 19:1, 2007.
- Koh BH et al; A Study on the Correlation of Metabolic Syndrome and Intima-media Thickness of Common Carotid Artery with Sasang Constitution, J Sasang Constitute Med, 2007.

- Koh BH et al; The Study on Sasangin's Appearance and Eating Habit of Elementary School Students, J Sasang Constitute Med, 2007.
- Koh BH et al; A Study on the Validity of the Questionnaire about Sasang Constitution Classification for Mongolians, J Sasang Constitute Med, 19:1, 2007.
- Koh BH et al; A Case Study about Soyangin Patient Suffering from Dizziness, Treated with Soyangin 'Exterior Cold Disease', J Sasang Constitute Med, 2007.
- Koh BH et al; An Error Analysis of the 3D Automatic Face Recognition Apparatus (3D-AFRA) Hardware, J Sasang Constitute Med, 2007.
- Koh BH et al; An Hardware Error Analysis of 3D Automatic Face Recognition Apparatus(3D-AFRA) Surface Reconstruction, J Sasang Constitute Med, 2007.
- Koh BH et al; A Case of Advanced Non-seminomatous Germ Cell Tumor of the Testis Cancer with Retroperitoneal Lymph Node Metastasis : Neoplastic Pain & Neoplastic Fever Treated by Sasang Constitutional Medical Treatment, J Sasang Constitute Med, 2007.
- Koh BH et al; A Case-Control Study on Risk Factors of Obese Patients of Each Sasang Constitution, J Sasang Constitute Med, 2007.
- Koh BH et al; A Case Of Symptoms and Quality Of Life Changes in Stage IV Gallbladder Cancer with Hematogenous Lung Metastasis by Sasang Constitutional Medicine, J Sasang Constitute Med, 2007.
- Koh BH et al; Development of Sasangin Diagnosis Questionnaire for School Aged Children, J Sasang Constitute Med, 2007.
- Koh BH et al; Clinical diagnosis and information on the Sasang apologetic for the senses sensor health monitoring system based on constitutional development, knowledge building, KIOM, 2007.
- Koh BH et al; A Software Error Examination of 3D Automatic Face Recognition Apparatus (3D-AFRA): Measurement of Facial Figure

Data, J Sasang Constitute Med, 2007.

- Koh BH et al; A Case of Stomach Cancer Patient with Peritoneum and Colon Metastasis Treated with Taeumjowi-tang for Abdominal Pain and Diarrhea, J Sasang Constitute Med, 2007.
- Koh BH et al; Development of Mongolian's SDQ (SDQ-M): Revision and Translation, J Sasang Constitute Med, 2007.
- Koh BH et al; A Study on the Facial Morphologic Characteristics of Mongolian according to Sasangin : Pilot Study, J Sasang Constitute Med, 2007.
- Koh BH et al; The Study on the Actual Nutrient Intake Based on Sasang Constitution, J Sasang Constitute Med, 19:3, 2007.
- Jung-Hee Yoo, Byung-hee Koh et al : Sasangin Diagnosis Questionnaire: Test of Reliability, J. of Alternative and Complimentary Medicine, 13:1 pp.111-122, 2007.
- Koh BH et al; The Upgrade of Sasangin Classification System by the Morphologic Study of Head and Face: Facial Differences on Sex and Age, J Sasang Constitute Med, 2007.
- Koh BH et al; A Case of Cervical Cancer Case with Urinary Disorder and Urticaria Managed by Sasang Constitutional Medicine, J Sasang Constitute Med, 2007.
- Lee JH, Kim YH, Hwang MW, Koh BH et al; Survey Study about Sasangin's Characteristics of Face, Voice, Skin and Pulse Diagnosis, J Sasang Constitute Med, 2007.
- Koh BH et al; A Study on the Mongolian's Morphologic Characteristics of face according to Sasang Constitution ; Pilot test, The 7th International Congress of Constitutional Medicine, 2007.
- Koh BH et al; Translation and Reliability Test of Mongolian's SDQ, The 7th International Congress of Constitutional Medicine, 2007.
- Koh BH et al; DB build for 3D constitutional diagnostic development (3rd year), KIOM, 2008.
- Koh BH et al; Accuracy of 3D Automatic Face Recognition Apparatus (3D-AFRA) Recognition, J Sasang Constitute Med, 2008.

- Koh BH et al; A Study on the Clinical Characteristics of Atopic Dermatitis According to Sasang Constitutions, J Sasang Constitute Med, 2008.
- Koh BH et al; The Study on the Formative Process of Taeumin's Dry-febrile Symptom, J Sasang Constitute Med, 2008.
- Koh BH et al; Practical methods of personalized medicine in accordance with the constitution, 2008 7th Sasang constitutional medicine Summer Conference symposium, 2008.
- Koh BH et al; A case study of a Somatoform Disorder Patient Diagnosed with Soyangin Symptomatic Pattern of 'Yin-Deficiency – Midday-Fever', J Sasang Constitute Med, 2008.
- Koh BH et al; A Study on Quality of Life of Advanced Hepatobiliary and Pancreatic Cancer patients Administered with Traditional Korean Cancer Treatment, J Korean Oriental Med, 2008.
- Koh BH et al; Base Research for the standard diagnosis of Sasang Medicine, KIOM, 2008.
- Koh BH et al; Studies on correlation with metabolic syndrome and glucose metabolism, hyperlipidemia, carotid IMT in taeeumin, - Preliminary Study, Kyunghee University, 2008.
- Koh BH et al; A Study on Dongmu's Thoughts about the Eight Items of "The Great Learning (Ta hsueh)", J Sasang Constitute Med, 2008.
- Koh BH et al; A Literature Study on the Concept and Classification of Soeumin Janggyeol, J Sasang Constitute Med, 2008.
- Koh BH et al; A Study of Soyangin's Delirious Speaking Bad Disease in Exterior Cold Disease induced from the Spleen Affected by Cold, J Sasang Constitute Med, 2008.
- Koh BH et al; The Study for Comparing between Theory about "Constitution" in Chinese Medicine and Sasang Constitutional Medicine in Korea, J Sasang Constitute Med, 2008.
- Koh BH et al; The Study of Sasangin's Face by the Items of Impression, J Sasang Constitute Med, 20:3, 2008.

- Koh BH et al; A Comparative Study of "HamsanSachon DongyiSuseBowon GaboGubon" and "SangGyoHyeonTo DongyiSuseBowon", J Sasang Constitute Med, 2008.
- Koh BH et al; Studies on absorption distribution and metabolism of ginseng in humans after oral administration, journal of ethno-pharmacology, Elsevier Ireland, 2008.
- Koh BH et al; 2005 sasangin diagnosis questionnaire for Mongolian (05`SDQ-M): test of reliability, The journal of alternative and complementary medicine, 2008.
- Koh BH et al; Acupuncture au Centre Medical de l'Universite Kyung Hee de Seoul, Coree-du-Sud, Acupuncture & Moxibustion, Meridiens, 7:4, 2008.
- Koh BH et al; A Literature Study on the Concept and Classification of Soyangin Gochang, J Sasang Constitute Med, 2009.
- Koh BH et al; A Sasang Constitutional Study on the Myunghyun Symptom, J Sasang Constitute Med, 2009.
- Yoo JH, Lee EJ, Koh BH et al; Test-Retest Method on Short Form Sasang Classification Questionnaire for American (SF_SSCQ-A): Pilot Study, J Sasang Constitute Med, 21:1, 2009.
- Koh BH et al; The Study on the Chronical Concept of Etiology in Sasang Constitutional Medicine (SCM), J Sasang Constitute Med, 21:1, 2009.
- Koh BH et al; A Case Study of 1 Taeeumin Patient Experiencing Hand Tremor, Heat Flash, and Dysarthria Treated Successfully with Yeoldahansotang, J Sasang Constitute Med, 2009.
- Koh BH et al; The Study for Comparing between Theory about "Constitution" in Chinese Medicine and Sasang Constitutional Medicine in Korea, J Sasang Constitute Med, 2009.
- Koh BH et al; The Study on Clinical Characteristics of Taeeumin Dry-Heat Symptomatic Patten, J Sasang Constitute Med, 2009.
- Koh BH et al; Odds Ratio of Dyslipidemia for Different Sasang Constitutional Types in Different BMI Groups, East-West interna-

tional multidisciplinary symposium, Kyunghee University Medical Center, 2009.

- Koh BH et al; Donguibogam Dongyi Suse Bowon, Donguibogam world record heritage values, KIOM, Donguibogam Memorial Consortium, 2009.
- Koh BH et al; Practical approach for tailored medicine based on Sasang constitution, Sasang Medicine personalized medicine, The Society of Sasang Constitutional Medicine, 2009.
- Koh BH et al; 2005 Sasang Classification Questionnaire for Mongolian: Test of Reliability, Sasang Medicine personalized medicine, The Society of Sasang Constitutional Medicine, 2009 / J. of Alternative and Complementary Medicine, 15:2, 2009, pp.165~174.
- Koh BH et al; Concept Analysis of Sasang Constitution: Application of Hybrid Model, The Society of Sasang Constitutional Medicine, 2009.
- Koh BH et al; Perspective of the Human Body in Sasang Constitutional Medicine, The Society of Sasang Constitutional Medicine, 2009.
- Koh BH et al; Literature on the use and origin of hyeongbang paedoksan, Sasang Medicine personalized medicine, The Society of Sasang Constitutional Medicine, 2009.
- Koh BH et al; The Study on The Origin, Changes, and Composition of Galgeulhaegi-tang, J Sasang Constitute Med, 21:2, 2009.
- Koh BH et al; A Pilot Study for the Construction of Sasang - Constitutionally Differentiated Model of the Metabolic Syndrome with Focus on 40~49 year old Taeumin, J Sasang Constitute Med, 2009.
- Koh BH et al; Reconsideration about the Dong-Mu's Theory of Nature and Emotion, J Sasang Constitute Med, 21:2, 2009.
- Hwang MW, Koh BH et al; The Study on the Pathology of Soeumin in Sasang Constitutional Medicine (SCM), J Sasang Constitute Med, 2009.

- Koh BH et al; The Origin, Change of the time and Constructive principle of Taeumjowitang, J Sasang Constitute Med, 2009.
- Koh BH et al; A Case Study of 1 Soyangin patient with sequence of Adult type Still's disease who reported symptomatic improvement after being treated with Hyeongbangjihwang-tang, J Sasang Constitute Med, 2009.
- Koh BH et al; Perspective of the Human Body in Sasang Constitutional Medicine, Evidence-based Complementary and Alternative Medicine, Oxford Journals, 2009.
- Koh BH et al; Sasang Constitution as a Risk Factor for Diabetes Mellitus: A Cross-Sectional Study, Evidence-based Complementary and Alternative Medicine, Oxford Journals, 2009.
- Koh BH et al; Anthropometric Facial Characteristics of Adult Taeeumin of Northern and Southern Lineage in the Korean Peninsula, The Journal of Korean medicine, 2009.
- Koh BH et al; The Study on the Pathology of Soyangin in Sasang Constitutional Medicine (SCM), J Sasang Constitute Med, 2009.
- Koh BH et al; Constitutional Health Care in Sasang Medicine, The 15th International Congress of Oriental Medicine (Program & Abstracts), ISOM, 2010.
- Koh BH et al; Sasangchejilgwa Limsangpyeolam, Hanmi medicine, 2010.
- Yoo JH, Shin HS, Lee JH, Lee EJ, Koh BH et al; The Item Analysis of Short Form Sasang Classification Questionnaire for American according to Comparison of Responses between Different Ethnic Groups: Pilot test, The Journal of Korean medicine, 2010 / J Sasang Constitute Med, 22:1, 2010.
- Koh BH et al; A case-control study on the risk factors for obesity across different sasang constitutional types, 5th international congress on complementary medicine research Abstract book, 2010.
- Koh BH et al; Two Cases of Repetitive Episodic Tension-type Headache Patients who were Constitutionally Typed as Soyangin

and Taeeumin, J Sasang Constitute Med, 2010.

- Koh BH et al; Theories on the Covetous Desire in the Quaternary Paradigm of Heaven-Human-Nature-Course within 「Donguisusebowon」 Theories on Nature and Conduct, J Sasang Constitute Med, 2010.
- Koh BH et al; Theories on the Covetous Desire in the Quaternary Paradigm of Heaven-Human-Nature-Course within 「Donguisusebowon」 Theories on Nature and Conduct, J Sasang Constitute Med, 2010.
- Koh BH et al; A Case Study Reporting Successful Treatment using Hyeongbangjihwang-tang of a Soyangin Patient diagnosed with Benign Arrhythmia and Experiencing Palpitation Symptoms, J Sasang Constitute Med, 2010.
- Koh BH et al; Sasang study of the clinical status, 14th Korea-China Conference symposium, Association of Korean Medicine, 2010
- Koh BH et al; Clinical Guideline of Operation for Constitutional syndrome, 14th Korea-China Conference symposium, Association of Korean Medicine, 2010.
- Koh BH et al; An Analysis of Eating Behaviors in Normal-Weight Males across Different Sasang Constitutional Types, J Sasang Constitute Med, 2010.
- Koh BH et al; Usages of Aconite, J Sasang Constitute Med, 2010.
- Koh BH et al; A Study on the Pathology and Therapeutics of Epigastric Discomfort in the Soeumin Taeum Symptomatology, J Sasang Constitute Med, 2010.
- Koh BH et al; The Origin, Changes and Compositive Principles of Hyangsayangyi-tang, J Sasang Constitute Med, 2010.
- Koh BH et al; Sasang Constitutional types can acts as a risk factor for insulin resistance, Diabetes Research and Clinical Practice, 2010.
- Koh BH et al; Sasang Constitutional types can acts as a risk factor for Hypertension, Clinical and Experimental Hypertension, 33:8, 2011.
- Koh BH et al; Comparison of sasang constitutional medicine, traditional Chinese medicine and Ayurveda. EVIDENCE-BASED

COMPLEMENTARY AND ALTERNATIVE MEDICINE, Hindawi Publishing Corporation, 2011.

- Koh BH et al; A discussion on the philosophical associations between Dongmu and Nosa: an approach based on the Li-Qi theory, J Sasang Constitute Med, 2011.
- Koh BH et al; A Study on the Therapeutic Herbal Medications for Soyangin Mangeum Symptomatology, J Sasang Constitute Med, 2011.
- Shin SW, Lee EJ, Lee JH, Koh BH et al; Study on the Development of Diagnosis Algorithm of Soeumin Symptomology, J Sasang Constitute Med, 2011.
- Koh BH et al; A study on the schematic organization of the sub-classification system of the Taeeumin symptomatology, J Sasang Constitute Med, 2011.
- Koh BH et al; Sasang Constitutional Types can Act as a Risk Factor for Insulin Resistance, The 9th International Congress of Sasang Constitutional Medicine, Abstract, J Sasang Constitute Med, KIOM, 2011.
- Koh BH et al; Sasang constitutional Types can Act as a risk factor for obesity and abdominal adiposity: A Cross-sectional study, The 9th International Congress of Sasang Constitutional Medicine, Abstract, J Sasang Constitute Med, KIOM, 2011.
- Koh BH et al; Short Form Sasang Classification Questionnaire for Mongolian (SF_SSCQ-M): Test of Reliability, the 9th International Congress of Sasang Constitutional Medicine, Abstract, Sasang Constitute Med, KIOM, 2011.
- Koh BH et al; Studies on Absorption, Distribution and Metabolism of Ginseng in Human after Oral Administration, The 9th International Congress of Sasang Constitutional Medicine, Abstract, Sasang Constitute Med, KIOM, 2011.
- Koh BH et al; The Origin, Changes and Compositive Principles of Baekhaoleejung-tang, J Sasang Constitute Med, 2011.

- Koh BH et al; The Origin, Changes and Compositive Principles of Yangkyuksanhwa-tang, J Sasang Constitute Med, 2011.
- Koh BH et al; The Origin, Change of the Time and Constructive Principle of Insamjinpi-tang, J Sasang Constitute Med, 2011.
- Koh BH et al; Approaching obesity through constitutional therapy: a series of 4 obesity cases who were classified as the Taeum constitutional type, J Sasang Constitute Med, 2011.
- Koh BH et al; A Study of Korean's Face by Sasang Diagnosis Using Questionnaire and 3D AFRA(Automatic Face Recognition Apparatus) in Middle Aged Women, J Sasang Constitute Med, 2011.
- Koh BH et al; Sasang Constitutional Medicine, Department of Health and Human Services, KIOM, 2011.
- Koh BH et al; Study on the Development of Diagnosis Algorithm of Soyangin Symptomatology, J Sasang Constitute Med, 2011.
- Koh BH et al; The influence of accumulated clinical experience with Soyang-type patients on the conceptualization of the Soyang pathology, J Sasang Constitute Med, 2011.
- Koh BH et al; An Analysis of Subjective Appetite Ratings across Different Sasang Constitutional Types, J Sasang Constitute Med, 2012.
- Koh BH et al; The Origin, Change, and Composition of Soeumin's Bojungikgi-tang, J Sasang Constitute Med, 2012.
- Koh BH et al; Comparison of Sasang constitutional medicine, traditional Chinese medicine and Ayurveda, The 1st annual academic conference of the specialty Committee of Constitutional medicine of WFCMS, WFCMS, 20120823.
- Koh BH et al; Diagnosis Algorithm of Soeumin Disease Pattern in Sasang Constitutional Medicine, 2012 Congress of Sasang Constitutional Medicine, Sasang Constitute Med, 2012.
- Koh BH et al; Suggestion of new possibilities in approaching individual variability in appetite through constitutional typology: a pilot study, BMC Complimentary and Alternative Medicine 2012.

- Koh BH et al; A Case study of Taeumin Esophagus Cold Pattern Patients with Gastro-esophageal Reflux Disease(GERD) and Irritable Bowel Syndrome(IBS), J Sasang Constitute Med, 2012.
- Koh BH et al; The Study on the Clinical Meanings of Ordinary Symptoms and Developing Aspects of Present Symptoms according to the Ordinary Symptoms in the Soeumin Symptomatology, J Sasang Constitute Med, 2012.
- Koh BH et al; The Methodological Review on the Accuracy Study of Questionnaire for Sasang Constitution Diagnosis, J Sasang Constitute Med, 2012.
- Koh BH et al; Development of Clinical Practice Guidelines for Sasang Constitutional Medicine Symptomatology-Purpose, Development Strategy and Procedure -, J Sasang Constitute Med, 2013.
- Koh BH; Sasang Constitutional Health Care System in Korea, 8thICTAMConference, 20130911.
- Koh BH, The Identity of Korean Medicine – focusing on Dr.Heo Jun and Dr. Lee, Jema, 20131009.
- Song EY, Lee EJ, Koh BH et al; The Study for standardized Method of the Retention-Enema; For a Method of Experimental Study: J Sasang Constitute Med, 2013.
- Koh BH et al; Association between Sasang Constitution, Impaired Lung Function and Metabolic Syndrome among Middle-aged Adults in Korea, J Sasang Constitute Med, 2013.
- Lee EJ, Koh BH et al; Clinical Practice Guideline for Soeumin Disease of Sasang Constitutional Medicine: Diagnosis and Algorithm: J Sasang Constitute Med, 26:1, 2014.
- Koh BH et al; Review of experimental and clinical studies on Soyangin Yanggyeoksanhwa-tang, oriental pharmacy and experimental medicine, springer, 2014.
- Lee EJ, Koh BH et al; Clinical Practice Guideline for Soyangin Disease of Sasang Constitutional Medicine: Overview, J Sasang Constitute Med, 2014.

- Koh BH et al; The Sasang Constitutional Types can act as a Risk Factor for Hypertension, 2015 ICCMR proceeding, 2015.
- Koh BH et al; Scientific Approach for Diagnosis of Tailored Medicine based on Constitution, The 12th World Congress of Chinese Medicine OBOR TCM CULTURE WEEK Abstracts o Conference Proceedings, World Federation of Chinese Medicine Societies, 2015.
- Koh BH et al; A study on the Conception of Ordinary Symptoms in Sasang Constitution Medicine, Conference Proceedings, World Federation of Chinese Medicine Societies, 20151128.
- Koh BH et al; Sasang Constitutional Medicine, Korean Medicine: Current Status and Future Prospects, Pusan National University College of Korean Medicine, pp.37-55, 2015, ISBN 978-89-969318-7-4.
- Koh BH et al; Clinical Practice Guideline for Taeeumin and Taeyangin Disease of Sasang Constitutional Medicine: Overview, J Sasang Constitute Med, 2014.
- Koh BH; Clinical applications of Sasang Constitutional Medicine: Shinjin Communications, Pusan National University College of Korean Medicine, Current Practice of Korean Medicine, pp.69-97, 2016.12.31., ISBN 979-11-88027-01-9.
- Lee EJ, Koh BH et al; Modification Principle of Taeeumjowi-tang in Sasang Medicine: J. of Sasang Constitute Med, pp. 215-224, 2016.09.30.
- Koh BH et al; The policy status of traditional medicine standardization between Korea and China as well as to derive a strategic development plan for Korean medicine standardization: J. of Korean Medicine, pp.97-111, 2016.09.01.
- Koh BH et al; The reliability and validity of SDQ_S for standardization of sasang constitutional diagnosis by korean medicine Specialist, J Sasang Constitute Med, pp.110-122, 2016.06.30.
- Koh BH et al; A Study of conception of Sojeung(Ordinary symp-

toms): J Sasang Constitute Med, pp.19-26, 2016.03.31.

- Koh BH et al; A Clinical Case Report of Soyangin Female Patients with Flushing:): J. of Sasang Constitute Med, pp.381-395, 2016. 12.31.
- Koh BH et al; Suggestion for Insurance Guarantee Reinforcement in Sasang Constitutional Examination and Counselling: J. of Sasang Constitute Med, 29:4, pp.299-310, 2017.12.31.
- Koh BH et al; Health Policy and Prospect for Traditional Korean Medicine; Shanghai International Forum on Traditional Medicine, 2F Grand ballroom, Huating hotel, Shanghai, China, 2017.11.24
- Koh BH et al; The Outline and Prospect of Sasang Constitutional Medicine: The 6th Annual Academic Conference of Specialty Committee of Constitutional Medicine of WFCMS, Shenzhen, 2017.11.03.
- Kang MS, Oh JW, Yang SP, Koh BH et al; A Study about Psychological Counseling Methods for Mental Curing Classified by Sasang Constitution:): J. of Sasang Constitute Med,30:1, pp.43-49, 2018.03.31.

General Terms

A

Acupuncture based on constitution (體質針法) 54
alcohol (酒) 63
anxious (不安定之心) 47
anxious mind (懼心) 46
authority and power (權勢) 61
avoiding all alcohol (禁酒) 60

C

causes deficiencies in the lower body and excess in the upper body (下虛上實) 48
Cultivate oneself. Bring order to the family. Govern the country. Bring peace to all. (修身齊家 治國平天下) 63
cold stomach syndrome (胃寒病證) 48
constitutional illnesses (體質病證) 47
covetous desires (心慾) 43
covetous determination (恒心) 45
cowardly mind (怯心) 46

D

deficient heat (虛熱) 50
dense and tight (稠密) 48
desires (心慾) 45
determination (恒心) 43
distinct definitions of health (完實無病) 47
『Dongui』 3, 8
『Donguibogam』 6, 7, 8
『Donguisusebowon』 4, 6, 10, 12

E

Eumheo-oyeol symptomatic pattern (陰虛午熱證) 50

excess in the upper areas and deficiencies in the lower areas (上盛下虛) 49

excessive heat (實熱) 50

expensive materials (嬌奢) 60

extravagant overspending (驕奢) 61

F

favor (Dangyeo; 黨與) 61

fire (火) 48

fire heat (火熱) 50

G

geungan (勤幹) 60

greed (心慾) 27

greed (貪慾) 61

greeds (慾) 62

『Gyeok』 3

『Gyeokchigo』 10

H

heat (熱) 48

humanity, justice, propriety, and wisdom (仁義禮智) 62

Hyunggyeok-yeol symptomatic pattern (胸膈熱證) 50

I

idealists (理想家) 60

illness (病證) 47

inclination of mind (心慾) 62

inclination of the mind (心慾) 62

internal heat (內熱) 48

irrational mind (偏私之心) 46

K

kidneys (腎) 44

L

large kidneys and small spleens (腎大脾小) 52
Lee, Jema 3, 5, 6, 7, 8, 9, 10, 12, 13, 15, 17, 55, 62, 63
listening and seeing (聞見) 61
liver (肝) 44
lungs (肺) 44

M

materialistic mind (物慾之心) 46
medicine and food share origins (醫食同源) 57
Mind and body (心身) 55, 56
mind/nature (心性) 43
moderation (中庸) 60

N

nature (性品) 58
natures (性) 62
negative characteristic(偸逸之心) 47

O

only move forward, and do not move backwards (慾進而不慾退) 45

P

pain (腫痛) 49
palpitations (怔忡) 46
paradise (武陵桃源) 60
paraparesis (解㑊) 47, 49
personality (性質) 43
phlegm (痰飮) 51

power (權) 63
proclivity and capacity (性質材幹) 27, 45

Q

qi (氣運) 58

R

real purpose (恒心) 62
regurgitation (噎膈) 47, 49
replenish yin (補陰) 51
rudeness, shallowness, greed, and indolence (鄙薄貪懶) 62

S

Sasang (四象) 13
SE-type 22, 23, 25, 26, 34, 36, 37, 38, 39, 40
self-indulgence (放縱之心) 45
severe diseases (重病) 47
sex (色) 63
sexual desires (好色) 60
simplify and minimize their lives (簡約) 61
small (小; weak) 52
Soeum (SE) type (少陰人) 3, 12, 13, 14
Soeumin (少陰人) 58
Soyang (SY) type (少陽人) 3, 12, 13, 14
Soyangin (少陽人) 58
spiritually and physically (心身) 56
spleen (脾) 44
spleen and stomach (脾胃) 52
SY-type 12, 22, 24, 25, 29, 30, 37, 38

T

Taeeum (TE) type (太陰人) 3, 12, 13, 14
Taekuk acupuncture method (太極鍼法) 54
Taeumin (太陰人) 58

Taeyang (TY) type (太陽人) 3, 12, 13, 14
Taeyangin (太陽人) 58
TE-type 22, 25, 31, 32, 36, 38, 39
they always prefer to stay in without coming forth (慾處而不慾出) 46
they do not often see matters through to their conclusion (慾擧而不慾措) 46
they prefer to remain still without moving (慾靜而不慾動) 46
thoughts and actions (知行) 62
Tidal fevers (燥熱病證) 48, 50
TY-type 22, 23, 26, 27, 28, 31, 36, 37

U

unhealthy states (大病) 47
upper body (上體) 49
upsurge (逆上) 47
urgent mind (急迫之心) 45

V

visceral (臟器) 58

W

wealth (財) 63

Y

Yang (陽) 13
yang deficiency syndrome (陽虛病證) 48
Yin (陰) 13

Names of Prescriptions in English

A

Akebiae Caulis Anxiety-Free Decoction 182
Angelicae Decursivae Radix and Rehmanniae Radi Preparata Decoction 181
Angelicae Gigantis Radix and Cynanchi Wilfordii Radix Middle-Soothing Decoction 156
Arisaematis Rhizoma and Aucklandiae Radix Qi-Correcting Powder 173
Armeniacae Semen Upraising-Clearing Decoction 126
Artemisiae Capillaris Herba and Aconiti Lateralis Radix Preparata Decoction 163

C

Cimicifugae Rhizoma and Angelicae Dahuricae Radix Stomach-Regulating Decoction 125
Cimicifugae Rhizoma and Scutellariae Radix Stomach-Regulating Decoction 125
Cinnamomi, Aconiti, Agastachis, and Citri Unshius Middle-Regulating Decoction 158
Cnidii, Angelicae Gigantis, Allii Fistulosi, and Perillae Middle- Regulating Decoction 158
Coptidis Rhizoma and Rehmanniae Radix Preparata Decoction 182
Coptidis Rhizoma White-Draining Powder 180
Cynanchi Wilfordii Radi and Cinnamomi Cortex Middle-Regulating Decoction 160
Cynanchi Wilfordii Radix Middle-Regulating Decoction 159
Cynanchi Wilfordii Radix Noble Decoction 154
Cyperi Rhizoma Ten Wholesome Decoction 154

D

Dioscoreae Rhizoma Lung-Prime Tonifying Decoction 130

E

Eight-Flavor Polyporus Decoction 198
Empirical Stomach-Regulating Decoction 125
Empirical Upraising-Clearing Decoction 126
Ephedrae Herba Stomach-Regulating Decoction 125
Euphorbiae Kansui Radix Minor Powder 191

F

Fire-Lowering Rehmanniae Radix Preparata Decoction 182
Four Poria Powder 187

G

Ginseng Radix and Cinnamomi Cortex Decoction 157
Ginseng Radix and Cynanchi Wilfordii Radix Middle-Soothing Decoction 156
Ginseng-Emphasized Cinnamomi Cortex Middle-Regulating Decoction 158
Ginseng-Emphasized Eight-Element Decoction 154

H

Holotrichiae Vermis Toxin-Repelling Powder 128

I

ISchizonepetae Spica Intestine- Cooling Decoction 185

K

Kidney Qi Stomach-Regulating Decoction 125

L

Lee's Diaphragm-Cooling Powder 188
Lung Clearing and Liver Purging Decoction 128
Lung-Moistening Liver-Clearing Decoction 128

M

Moutan Cortex and Rehmanniae Radix Preparata Decoction 182
Myristicae Semen and Aconiti Lateralis Radix Preparata Middle-Regulating Decoction 159

N

Nine-Flavor Piteous Flower Decoction 152

P

Piteous Flower Rehmanniae Radix Preparata Decoction 188
Piteous Flower Stomach-Regulating Decoction 125
Puerariae Radix Major Qi-Coordinating Decoction 129
Puerariae, Cervi Parvum Cornu, and Spirodelae Decoction 131

Q

Qi-Coordinating Stomach-Regulating Decoction 125
Qi-Securing Stomach-Regulating Decoction 125

R

Raphani Semen Qi-Coordinating Decoction 129
Rehmanniae Radix Crudus et Preparata Decoction 182

S

Scrophulariae Radix and Rehmanniae Radix Preparata Decoction 182
Spirit relieving and Liver Purging Decoction 128
Stomach-Regulating Life-Prolonging Decoction 125

T

Ten Wholesome Greatly Tonifying Decoction 154
Three Spirit Powder 133
Three White Middle-Regulating Decoction 159
Trogopterorum Faeces Middle-Soothing Decoction 156
Twelve-Flavor Middle-Soothing Decoction 156

W

Warming and Transforming Pellet 157

Y

Yang-Restoring Greatly Tonifying Decoction 161
Yang-Upraising Eight-Element Decoction 154
Yellow-White Tiger Decoction 187

Z

Zingiberis Rhizoma and Atractylodis Rhizoma Alba
Middle-Soothing Decoction 156

Names of Prescriptions in Romanized Korean

A

Anhoe-san 148

B

Baekhaobujaijung-tang 159
Baekhaogunja-tang 154
Baekhaogwangyeijung-tang 160
Baekhaoijung-tang 159
Baekho-tang 187
Baekhoikwon-san 200
Baekhotang-go 200
Bakha-jeon 204
Bangpungtongseong-san 195
Bibanghwache-hwan 165
Boikgogi-tang 174
Bojungikgi-tang 152
Bomyeong-eum 167
Bopyetongyu-san 138
Bopyewon-tang 130
Botae-eum 139
Botaejihwang-tang 194
Bujaijung-tang 158
Bulsu-eum 168
Bupyeongdaehwang-tang 143
Byeokryeok-san 163

C

Chanhwa-dan 202
Cheongeumdojeok-san 196

Cheongeumjowi-tang 149
Cheongeummunmu-tang 137
Cheongpyesagan-tang 128
Cheongryangsanhwa-tang 199
Cheongsimsanyak-tang 143
Cheongsimyeonja-tang 127
Cheongunggyeji-tang 152
Cheonmundongyunpye-tang 142
Cheosaeng-san 191
Chilgi-tang 171
Chilmijeoryung-tang 198

D

Daebo-tang 161
Daegamsu-san 191
Daehwang-san 139
Daehwangjeogeunpi-tang 146
Danbaekho-tang 197
Dangguibaekhaogwanjung-tang 156
Dangguionjung-tang 178
Danggyul-tang 170
Dohaebaekho-tang 197
Dokhwaljihwang-tang 181
Doksamgwangyeijung-tang 158
Doksamijung-tang 176
Doksampalmul-tang 154
Doksamyangbung-tang 177
Donlan-san 191

G

Gagamcheongsim-tang 147
Galgeunbupyeong-tang 131
Galgeundaeseunggi-tang 129
Galgeunhaegi-tang 126

Galgeunseunggi-tang 129
Galyongbupyeong-tang 131
Gamgyul-jeon 171
Gamibaekho-tang 203
Gamicheongsim-tang 146
Gamihanso-tang 147
Gamijihwang-tang 202, 204
Gamijowi-tang 148
Gamipalmul-tang 172
Gamisanhwa-tang 203
Gamsucheonil-hwan 185
Gangbu-tang 160
Gangchulgwanjung-tang 156
Gangchulpajeok-tang 175
Gangeumbaekho-tang 193
Ganghwajihwang-tang 182
Geonbijangwi-tang 174
Geonyuljejo-tang 131
Geonyuljeogeunpi-tang 132
Geopunghaeeo-san 137
Geumsa-ju 169
Geumsangcheomhwabaekho-tang 197
Gilgyeong-tang 147, 149
Gilgyeongjeogeunpi-tang 143
Gilgyeongsaengmaek-san 142
Gogijowi-tang 125
Gondam-tang 136
Gongjinheugwon-dan 130
Guisinhaeeo-tang 192
Guisinilchalgwang 136
Gungguichongsoijung-tang 158
Gungguihyangso-san 153
Gwache-san 132
Gwakhyangjeonggi-san 173
Gwangyedoksampalmul-tang 175

Gwanjung-tang 159
Gyebugwakjinijung-tang 158
Gyegi-go 177
Gyeji-tang 160
Gyejibanhasaenggang-tang 155
Gyejibuja-tang 162
Gyejichongsoijung-tang 176
Gyeongbungamsujawung-dan 186
Gyeongbungamsuyongho-dan 186
Gyeongbunyuhyangmolyak-hwan 186
Gyeongheomseungcheong-tang 126
Gyeonghumjowi-tang 125
Gyeonjeong-san 170
Gyesam-go 156

H

Haegidaean-tang 141
Haenginmaekmundong-tang 145
Haenginseungcheong-tang 126
Handayeolso-tang 128
Heunno-hwan 134
Hoeyangdaebo-tang 161
Hwalseokgosam-tang 180
Hwangbaekho-tang 187
Hwanggigeyjibuja-tang 150
Hwanggigyeji-tang 152
Hwanggisoyeop-tang 174
Hwangryeoncheongjang-tang 185
Hwangryeonjeodu-tang 188
Hwangryeonjihwang-tang 182
Hwangryeonsabaek-san 180
Hwangyulgogi-tang 144
Hwangyulomija-go 144
Hwaseokjihwang-tang 188
Hwaseokjowi-tang 125

Hyangbujapalmul-tang 154
Hyangbusipjeon-tang 154, 155
Hyangsaijung-tang 176
Hyangsayangwi-tang 155
Hyangsayukgunja-tang 166
Hyangso-san 162
Hyeongbangdojeok-san 179
Hyeongbangjihwang-tang 181
Hyeongbangpaedok-san 179
Hyeongbangsabaek-san 180
Hyeonsambaekho-tang 193
Hyeonsampaedok-san 195
Hyunsamjihwang-tang 182

I

Ijung-tang 160
Imunomi-tang 138
Indongdeungjigolpi-tang 184
Injinbuja-tang 163
Injingyulpi-tang 163
Injinsayeok-tang 163
Insam-san 167
Insamaengsok-tang 177
Insambaekhaogwanjung-tang 156
Insamgeyjibuja-tang 150
Insamgwangyebuja-tang 151
Insamgyepi-tang 157
Insamjinpi-tang 157
Insamosuyu-tang 157
Iphyo-san 135
Iseonggugo-hwan 135
Issibia-hwan 189
Issidojeok-san 189

J

Jangdal-hwan 164
Jejopaedok-san 128
Jeokbaekhaogwanjung-tang 155
Jeoksa-jeon 167
Jeokseokjiuycoryang-tang 161
Jeoman-san 191
Jeonggicheonhyang-tang 171
Jeongsinsagan-tang 128
Jeonhojihwang-tang 181
Jeoryeong-tang 187
Jeoryeongbaekho-tang 198
Jeoryeongchajeonja-tang 180
Jihwang-tang 201
Jihwangbaekho-tang 182
Jihwanghyeonmu-tang 194
Jihwangpaedok-san 201
Jineum-hoe 166
Jogakdaehwang-tang 131
Jogaksamhwang-tang 143
Joripyewon-tang 129
Jowiseungcheong-tang 126
Jowisongmyung-tang 125
Jusaikwon-san 185

L

Leesiseunggi-tang 140
Leesiyanggyeok-san 188

M

Maekmundong-tang 144
Maekmundongwonji-san 133
Mahwangbalpyo-tang 129
Mahwanggeumsu-tang 141

Mahwangjeongcheon-tang 127
Mahwangjeongtong-tang 127
Mahwangjowi-tang 125
Mangeummunmu-tang 137
Mokdanjihwang-tang 182
Mokhyangsungi-san 161
Moktongdaean-tang 184
Moktonggosam-tang 199
Moktongmuwu-tang 182
Munmubotae-eum 140
Myeongmok-san 138

N

Naebokjaseunggi-tang 129
Nangan-san 169
Nokyongdaebo-tang 130
Nokyongdaejo-tang 142

O

Omae-jeon 149
Onbaek-won 164
Onhwa-dan 157
Onjung-eum 168
Oryeong-san 187
Oryeongjigwanjung-tang 156
Osuyubujaijung-tang 158

P

Padu-dan 157
Padu-go 172
Palmigosam-tang 198
Palmijeoryung-tang 198
Palmulgunja-tang 153
Pyojeungbaekho-tang 193

S

Saengjihwang-tang 189
Saengmaek-san 135
Saengsukjihwang-tang 182
Sahyang-san 132
Sain-san 173
Sambaekijung-tang 159
Samhwang-san 139
Samhwangseokin-san 148
Sammisamyu-tang 163
Sammulbaek-san 165
Samneungsojeok-hwan 164
Samsin-san 133
Sanmil-go 167
Sanmil-tang 156
Sanyakbopyewon-tang 130, 134
Saryeong-san 187
Sasi-dan 145
Sayeok-tang 160
Seokchangpowonji-san 133, 134
Seonghyangjeonggi-san 153, 173
Seunggeumjowi-tang 125
Seunggijowi-tang 125
Seungjijowi-tang 125
Seungmagaenoe-tang 141
Seungyangikgi-tang 151
Seungyangikgibuja-tang 150
Seungyangpalmul-tang 154
Sibimigwanjung-tang 156
Sibimijihwang-tang 182
Sihocheongbok-tang 200
Sihogwaru-tang 196
Sihosaryeong-tang 196
Sindaesiho-tang 192
Singi-hwan 187

Singijowi-tang 125
Sinsosiho-tang 192
Sipjeondaebo-tang 154
Sodok-eum 190
Sogamsu-san 191
Sohaphyang-won 162
Sojadodam-tang 178
Soyangbowi-tang 201
Subihaeeo-tang 170
Sueunhunbi-bang 190
Suhwagije-tang 199
Sukjihwanggosam-tang 184

T

Taeeumjowi-tang 125
Toehwang-eum 135
Tongyuguisin-tang 194

U

Uiinjowi-tang 146

W

Wuhwangcheongsim-hwan 133
Wuhwangsanyak-won 144
Wungdam-san 132

Y

Yangdokbaekho-tang 183
Yanggyeok-san 188
Yanggyeoksanhwa-tang 183
Yangui-jeon 203
Yeoldahanso-tang 128
Yeongsa-san 190

Yeosin-ju 136
Yeosin-tang 172
Yeoui-chim 168
Yeoui-dan 166
Yeoui-do 168
Yongyukjowi-tang 149
Yuhwang-san 169
Yuhyangmolyakgyeongbun-hwan 186
Yukdugubujaijung-tang 159
Yungmijihwang-tang 188
Yunpyecheonggan-tang 128